Michelangelo's Medicine

Michelangelo's Medicine

HOW REDEFINING THE HUMAN BODY WILL TRANSFORM HEALTH AND HEALTHCARE

Anoop Kumar, MD

© 2017 Anoop Kumar, MD
All rights reserved.

ISBN-13: 9780997339604
ISBN-10: 0997339608

The human body is the best picture of the human soul.
-LUDWIG WITTGENSTEIN

Table of Contents

Preface ································ix

Acknowledgements ·······················xiii

Part I: Redefining the Human Body and Transforming Health ········1

Chapter 1   What is the Future of Emergency Care? ··············3

Chapter 2   How did I Get Here? ··························9

Chapter 3   Two Worlds ································17

Chapter 4   Is Anatomy in the Eye of the Beholder? ············23

Chapter 5   What is Well-Being? ··························31

Chapter 6   Angel in the ED ····························41

Chapter 7   What are the Three Bodies? ····················49

Chapter 8   What are the Four Pillars? ····················67

Part II: Transforming Health Care ·············· 77

Chapter 9   State of the Medical System ············ 79

Chapter 10 What is the Informational Problem? ······· 87

Chapter 11 What is Energy? ····················· 99

Chapter 12 Why do we Need a Science of Well-Being? ······· 109

Chapter 13 What is the Next Step in the Evolution of Science? ···· 125

Chapter 14 What will Medical Training Look Like in the Future? ·· 139

Part III: How we Get There ·················· 145

Chapter 15 Dear Clinician ····················· 147

Chapter 16 A Declaration of Well-Being ············ 151

Chapter 17 A Blueprint for Well-Being ············· 155

Glossary ····························· 159

Preface

Michelangelo di Lodovico Buonarroti Simoni was born on March 6, 1475. Over a career spanning the better part of a century, he came to be known as one of the greatest artists who ever lived. Among his body of work are two of the most recognizable pieces in the world—*The Creation of Adam* on the ceiling of the Sistine Chapel and the statue of David. There were many great Renaissance artists, but Michelangelo was especially renowned for one reason: he created masterpieces.

In May 2016, I had the opportunity to take in some of this master's work during a visit to Florence, Italy, for a medical conference. I had seen many pictures of David and heard of his greatness, but I was curious to experience him in person. What surprised me most was not the anatomical detail of David but the personality and presence that radiated from the figure. Standing near him, one can feel his determination and poise. Beyond that, his sheer presence makes itself known. David is a sculpture of not just a physical body but a complete human being. This was Michelangelo's genius. He saw beyond the physical body and was able to reproduce that vision in marble.

I had already started writing a manuscript for this book prior to arriving in Florence. While there, I began to wonder, *how might Michelangelo envision and depict what we know about the human body today? What is the true masterpiece around which health and health care might revolve?* This was the inspiration for the title of this book.

Contemplating along these lines inspired me to move forward with the new model of the human being presented in this book. It also inspired me to reach further and sketch a broad and comprehensive vision of not just health but also health care and medical science. The way I saw it, I couldn't do justice to our understanding of the human being, of ourselves, without also addressing its applications; I couldn't leave the centerpiece without its limbs.

I wrote this book because the picture of health and health care that medical science paints is remarkably incomplete. That picture influences not only those within the health care system but everyone in our society. It is the knowledge we all subscribe to. That knowledge incompletely depicts a living, thinking, feeling, evolving human being—a true masterpiece— as a rigid, physical structure. As a result, too many people—patients, clinicians, and many others—are suffering unnecessarily.

The degree of incompleteness in medical science today cannot be acceptable in a modern society with the world's knowledge at its fingertips. Such incompleteness paves the way for innumerable people across the world to develop health emergencies and end up in emergency departments. What if some of the diseases we consider fatal are, in fact, curable? What if many lifelong battles against chronic diseases are avoidable? What if everyday life could be more enjoyable if we simply understood the human body more completely?

To begin converting these possibilities into realities, this book offers a way forward. That way forward includes not only healing and eliminating unnecessary suffering but also feeling the wonder we experience in the presence of a masterpiece. That masterpiece is you—the whole you.

I present this picture to you from my perspective as an emergency physician who sees life-threatening emergencies on a daily basis at work. I recognized that the stories we have been told about health, disease, and health care are just that—stories from one perspective. In this book, we will explore other, equally important, perspectives that have been either misunderstood or ignored altogether.

Each of the three parts of this book has a distinct feel. The theme in Part I, "Redefining the Human Body and Transforming Health," is how we can reconcile the different perspectives on the human body and experience the body anew. My approach is that of reflection and direct experience: How else might we *see* the body? What does the body *feel* like?

I didn't feel I could legitimately present the breadth of information covered in this book without offering you substantial insight into the experiences that inform my views, so I approached the above questions by offering accounts of my own explorations of the human body. Those insights are formulated into a complete model of the human being, called The Three Bodies, which I present at the end of Part I.

The theme in Part II, "Transforming Health Care," is how we can bring the complete experience of being human into a true health care system. Translating our direct experience into a science-based, practical system is a task that requires a strong conceptual framework. Accordingly, Part II is more analytical, beginning by focusing a spotlight on the core informational problem in health care that too few are talking about. A possible solution to the problem is then explored through an analysis of the nature of energy and information and how they may contribute to a science of well-being.

The theme in Part III, "How We Get There," is action. I list concrete steps we can take to further clarify our understanding and facilitate changes in our lives, in our communities, and in health care.

I suggest reading this book not only to glean information but to experience new aspects of yourself. I invite you to pause and contemplate new perspectives as they come up, even if (especially if) they may seem counterintuitive at first glance. This is the real value of this book.

Because some of the descriptions require us to view old concepts through a different lens, I've used common phrases in new ways throughout the book, in effect creating a new lexicon with the goal of a more precise, clutter-free understanding. Whenever I do this, I underline the phrase I'm using in a new way. Especially important concepts, such as that of a "healing system," are underlined throughout the text. Underlined phrases can be referenced in the Glossary, where I clarify their intended meaning. I've also tried to anticipate and address the most common doubts a reader may have in the Q&A section at the end of many chapters. These doubts reflect the ones I myself had along the way.

Ultimately, this book is not only about a vision of health. It's also about how we experience our lives, moment to moment. It's about finding a way to place a living masterpiece at the center of your immediate experience, as well as at the center of health and health care. We have the ability and the tools to accomplish this. Let us settle for nothing less.

Anoop Kumar, MD, MM

Acknowledgements

I cannot say that this book is the work of one person. Its soul has been forged by many. Foremost among them are Malini, Surya, Anjali, and the innumerable patients I've seen over the last ten years. Their patience, insight, and encouragement are woven through the pages of this book. For this, I offer my eternal gratitude.

To my patients in the emergency department, I have to say another word. Where would I be without you? How much less I would know of myself! It is my good fortune that you allow me into your private world to share your fear, anguish, and relief. To walk into a room and meet a fellow human being fearing the worst is a sacred experience that stirs the soul. No one walks away from that experience the same, whether for the first or thousandth time. By holding up a mirror to my soul, you guided me to the knowledge that the moment we live now is ever free, untouched by the shores of life and death. For this, I offer my eternal gratitude.

Part I
Redefining the Human Body and Transforming Health

Part I

CHAPTER 1
What is the Future of Emergency Care?

William had been trying to sleep for hours, but the gnawing pain in his chest was keeping him awake. Finally, when he started feeling nauseous, he got out of bed and headed for the medicine cabinet to grab his reflux pills. After sitting upright for the next forty-five minutes, trying to prevent the acid in his stomach from making its way up into his chest, he lay back down, only to find that he was sweating profusely.

His wife awoke and saw the discomfort on his face. She suggested that they see a doctor first thing in the morning. "I don't think I can wait that long," William gasped.

Within ten minutes an ambulance reached their home. The emergency medical technicians immediately placed a *vital-band* around William's elbow. The *vital-band* was a three-and-a-half-inch-long cuff that continuously sent real-time information on William's blood pressure, heart rate, oxygen level, and temperature to the ambulance's monitor, as well as to the off-site emergency physician serving as medical control for the county. With each heartbeat, a new set of vitals appeared:

Blood pressure	168/88
Heart rate	90
Respiratory rate	22
Oxygen saturation	96%
Temperature	99.0

Like all health care personnel, the ambulance crew had undergone extensive training in meditative techniques. They understood that the way they communicated and interacted with the patient had the ability to sustain the disease process or begin to heal it. As they laid a *bio-skin* over William's clothes, their breathing cadence was measured and deliberate, influencing the patient's own breathing.

The *bio-skin* looked very similar to a cloth sheet from 2016. It extended from William's neck to his knees and from one arm to the other. No sooner had they laid it atop him than an electrocardiogram and a live video of the heart, lungs, and abdominal organs appeared on their monitor, the remote physician's monitor, and the closest emergency department's data center.

The electrocardiogram was suggestive of a non-ST elevation myocardial infarction—a type of heart attack. The real-time movie did not show any major abnormalities. The heart seemed to be pumping appropriately without any distortion of its compartments, the lungs were expanding and contracting as they should, and there was no sign of abdominal obstruction or injury.

In the meantime, the *vital-band* had ultrasonically located a vein, secreted a sterile local anesthetic, painlessly placed an intravenous catheter, and drawn two milliliters of blood. The results of the blood tests would be reported momentarily.

William felt he was in good hands. The medical crew was calm and capable, moving efficiently—not a movement out of place, not a motion wasted—as if the scene had been choreographed and practiced over and over. They explained to William and his wife what they were doing, even as they moved quickly and quietly, one action flowing into the next. William felt he could trust them.

The crew slipped a sturdy yet malleable half-inch-thick *transporter* under William as he lay in the bed. Holding it by the front, they led it forward and down the stairs with William aboard. One crew member gently placed his hand on William's chest and let it remain there as they moved him, immediately calming his nerves. The crew easily maneuvered the support panel; it only took the slightest tug from a single finger to move it.

By the time William reached the ambulance, energetic treatment had already been initiated: the *vital-band* vibrated at a particular frequency that helped the patient relax, and its ambient light adjusted to a particular frequency of blue known to inhibit the activity of myofilaments in the blood vessels that supply the heart. When myofilament activity decreases, the muscles in the vessel walls relax and the vessels open up, increasing blood flow to critical areas of the heart.

The *bio-skin* showed that the initial changes on the electrocardiogram were now reverting to normal. William's chest pain was gone. The crew member removed his hand from William's chest. William's breathing was deep and deliberate. His vital signs now read:

Blood pressure	133/79
Heart rate	72
Respiratory rate	10
Oxygen saturation	99%
Temperature	98.8

In the past, the crew would have used nitroglycerin to open up the blood flow to the heart. It was a powerful agent, but in certain types of heart attacks and in some patients taking other medications, it could precipitously drop blood pressure and worsen the patient's clinical condition. Frequency therapy had the effect of interacting with the Energetic Body in such a way as to lower the blood pressure safely while maintaining proper blood flow to the organs.

By the time William reached the emergency department (ED), the blood tests were complete and supported the diagnosis of a minor heart attack. William had no remaining symptoms. The necessary medications had already been prepared in the exact dosage needed, taking into account William's weight, which the *transporter* had transmitted to the hospital when William was being loaded into the ambulance.

Within seventeen minutes of William's arrival in the ED, the emergency physician had evaluated William's clinical status, medications had been administered, and the diagnosis had been finalized. Now the next phase of treatment began. A second clinician came into the room, introduced herself, and began to chat with William. After a brief conversation, she picked up his left hand and held it face-up in her own left hand. Using the index and middle fingers of her right hand, she felt for the pulsations of his radial artery near the wrist. She closed her eyes and held this position for approximately two minutes—no questions, no movements.

William detected that she was using her fingers deftly to check how his pulse was responding to external pressure. Sometimes she pressed deeply and maintained pressure; at other times she applied a quick pulse of pressure, checking to see how the vessel rebounded. When she was done, there was no detailed conversation about what she had learned. Instead, she informed William that the most important thing for him to do in this moment was rest. The information she gleaned about the constitution of his Three Bodies would be noted and reviewed with him the next day to create a health map.

As William was being moved to his room, he noticed that each of the rooms in the ED had a different hue. He saw an anxious and screaming patient become calm within seconds of being touched in the middle of his chest. William couldn't hear it, but audio speakers in each room were also playing sound patterns unique to each room and audible only within that room, influencing The Three Bodies of the unique patient in that room.

William's wife noted that when the ED was full, newly arriving patients waited in one of three healing rooms if they were not critically ill. Each healing room was emitting light and sound frequencies that balanced a particular constitution of The Three Bodies. By the time these patients reached their treatment rooms, the healing process had already begun and could be further customized for the individual by the treating physician.

Replacing the waiting room with healing rooms had a dramatic effect on the ED. Patients who had to wait to see a physician were usually not agitated, anxious, or upset—their problems were already being addressed. This made the clinical staff calmer and the overall atmosphere more pleasant and conducive to healing.

Patients who were well enough to go home after treatment received information about how their illness manifested in each of their Three Bodies, with recommendations for treatment of each body. They could go online to the international health database to see how each healing system approached their illness and treated each of The Three Bodies. Because many of the most powerful treatments for the Energetic and Mental Bodies were either free or inexpensive, patients were able to actively manage their own well-being, with health practitioners guiding them along the way.

Since the time William had worked in the ED as a nurse twenty years prior, the number of visits to the ED for exacerbations of chronic disease had plummeted. He ascribed this not only to a more complete understanding of the human body but also to the recognition that well-being was about more than keeping the Physical Body going at any cost.

The revolution in well-being over the last couple decades had spilled over from popular culture to medical science, as scientists began shifting their perspectives on not only their research but themselves as well. People were recognizing and exploring aspects of themselves that they had never known existed before.

The cost of end-of-life care had been cut in half, as people were placing a premium on overall well-being. Patients were happier because they were being seen as whole persons, not just physical bodies with symptoms of disease. They no longer had to squeeze their subjective experiences of well-being, including their feelings and intuition, into a story about physical symptoms.

The clinical staff were happier because they had a more complete understanding of the person behind the patient. They understood which of The Three Bodies they were trained to address, and they were able to arrange for a variety of approaches to healing guided by a range of health practitioners based on what might work best for each unique patient. They developed this knowledge within a model of interprofessional learning during their medical education, also gaining a direct appreciation for what well-being is and how it can be developed. Administrators were happy because patients were happy, staff turnover was low, and most departments were regularly collecting bonuses for keeping the surrounding population healthy.

As he thought back to his career in the ED, William could still hear the loud, disruptive noises, see the anxious patients and staff, and feel the incessant race against time to manage every patient with a one-size-fits-all model of care. He remembered how nobody understood the relationship between frequencies of light and sound and how the Energetic Body functioned; how the light used in the main work area and patient rooms created anxiety in the human nervous system; how nobody thought to use technology to transform noise into healing sound; how few recognized the technology behind touch; and how the Mental and Energetic Bodies were considered either mythical or inaccessible. "We were working against ourselves and we didn't even realize it," he mused. "We were in the dark ages."

William remembered how the placebo effect was weeded out of medical care in the old days. Since that time, the understanding of the placebo effect had evolved from the idea that it was a random event, to an understanding that belief could have an unpredictable effect, to the realization that intention could result in a reproducible effect, and ultimately to the knowledge that molding our bodies was a learnable skill. "People would've never believed this was possible back when I was working in the ED," chuckled William.

No longer did doctors tell patients that their expected five-year survival rate for a particular condition was only 20 percent. They had learned that repeating such a statistic only made it more likely that a negative result would occur—the nocebo effect. They had learned that they couldn't possibly predict which person would recover from an illness at what time and for what reason. They could only make general predictions across large populations, never specifically for the patient in front of them. Because of a combination of understanding the human body more completely, focusing on well-being, developing new energetic and mental therapeutics, and avoiding nocebo effects while harnessing the placebo effect, cancer was now a disease of the last generation.

William had just had a heart attack, but seeing how far health care had come brought a smile to his face.

CHAPTER 2
How did I Get Here?

I often get asked how I, a practicing emergency physician, became so interested in the big picture beyond the ED. Doesn't the fact that I am an emergency physician mean that I'm supposed to fix immediate problems and not dwell on that "big picture"? Yes, I suppose it does, to a large extent, but what happens when it's the big picture itself that's creating the immediate problems?

During my emergency medicine training, it was clear to me that my role was like a firefighter's—putting out a series of medical fires as quickly as possible. It's a critical job, one that defines the ED, but I couldn't shake the disquieting feeling that the primary interest of the medical treatment system was "fire management," and little more. The system's approach to the health of our patients, or rather to their illnesses, felt superficial.

It seemed obvious that the lives of too many people were enduring long-term harm from this institutional focus on the immediate "quick fix." Too many people were, and are, suffering. The *people* that I refer to were not just patients but clinicians as well.

When speaking about how to improve the medical treatment system, many experts tend to divide patients from clinicians, addressing each group separately. But from what I've seen, the root cause of suffering is the same for both groups.

Medical training has little to do with health. Physicians don't study health. We don't study human beings in their entirety. We study disease processes. Accordingly, our working environments, practices, and medical treatment system as a whole aren't designed to support health, despite our best efforts.

Is it any wonder the physician suicide rate in the United States is *twice* the nonphysician rate, or that "burnout" among nurses is causing dangerously high turnover rates? Is it any wonder patients with chronic illness repeatedly suffer painful relapses, month after month, year after year? We live with the expectation that health care should foster health. We hold on to that possibility (and we should) even as we settle for beating back disease, one episode at a time.

This assessment made me very uncomfortable. I had spent many years learning medicine. I am proud of serving as an emergency physician, doing whatever possible to help another person in a time of need. The problems that I now perceived in the medical treatment system threatened the image I had of myself as a doctor.

I felt like I had to choose sides between what I had been taught then and what I was learning now from my own experiences. I could see my fellow physicians and nurses also struggling to adapt our one-dimensional training to our real-life, multidimensional patients. I could see the suffering this caused everyone, but I didn't know what to do about it. I was caught between the medical treatment system I was working in and the healing system I knew without a doubt was possible.

My mind was divided, and that division kept me doubting whether my interpretations were correct. It kept me within the codified groupthink of the medical treatment system. So, when I saw a patient having a heart attack, I believed that if only he could make it to the catheterization lab in time, then a perfectly placed stent would solve the problem. When I saw a patient with recurrent asthma, I believed that if only she had medical insurance, she would be able to get her medication regularly and be just fine. And when I saw a patient with an episode of severe pain, I believed that if only he was able to keep his scheduled appointments with his care specialists, together they could develop a plan to manage the pain, or maybe even cure it. While getting a stent placed, having medical insurance, or seeing your physician regularly are obviously important, they only partially address the problems plaguing our medical treatment system.

I began to dig deeper, listening to many experts, reading many books, and having many conversations. I soon recognized that while politics and profit contribute to many systemic problems, lurking beneath these issues was an even more basic problem: the lack of a full understanding of the nature of the human being.

I hesitated at this point. It seemed that the more I tried to get to the bottom of the troubled American medical treatment system, the bigger the challenge became. I could see why the simpler fixes suggested for "health care reform" were the norm. To talk about what is needed to create a true health care system is too complex, too politically and personally risky, too "radical."

Though I had many doubts, my investigation didn't stop. I was seeing so many patients in the ED with acute, life-threatening illnesses, with many more returning due to chronic problems, and my colleagues were burning out, one after the other. It got to the point where I couldn't just go through the motions anymore.

Although I was fulfilling my responsibilities as an ED doc, I found it increasingly difficult to shut out the troubling Big Picture. I wanted not just to work within my job description but also to advocate for the well-being of all patients, my colleagues, and the public at large. This was a responsibility I felt I had to fulfill.

When I discussed my observations with friends and colleagues, the most common response was, "You're right. We need to focus more on prevention. That's what's missing." Only that *wasn't* what was missing.

Surely, disease prevention must become a bigger priority in America, but that's just the point: preventing *disease* is still about *disease*. The medical treatment system views prevention as avoiding disease. The simplest example of this is the annual check-up, intended to prevent something serious from developing down the line. But surely there's more to health than running away from disease. We have to know more than that ... or at least we should.

Shouldn't we also be moving *toward* what is possible? This question of "what is possible?" is what truly intrigued me. Observing how clinical medicine was being practiced convinced me that the medical treatment system did not know what was possible. It was not aware of its own blind spot—the true nature of the human being and the true nature of health.

I was still apprehensive about taking this further. The challenges were growing. I wanted to throw in the towel. We all know what that feels like: looking deeply enough into a problem, seeing exactly what the nature of the beast is, and thinking *forget it, life's too short.*

But I couldn't give up, no matter how impossible things seemed. Ignoring objections from my rational mind, I started a blog, then another one, then yet another. The first blog was an inquiry into wellness—what it meant and what its implications were. The second was an exploration of the intersection of wellness and health care. The third iteration, which continues today at anoopkumar.com, went right to the heart of the matter—how to experience the masterpiece within you. Along the way, I started to see the relationship between health and the overall <u>medical treatment system</u> in a different light.

At first, I thought that politics and profits were at the heart of the system's many problems. (There's certainly an argument to be made for this.) But as I studied the problem, I saw that the most important part missing from my perspective was *us*—you and me.

This *us* is something that goes beyond the role of patient and physician to a more fundamental place, one where health care is about what's fundamental to all of us as human beings. I saw that I had to step out of the role of being a physician and question my own experience at a very basic level.

That's when I started to explore what health meant to me, what it *felt* like. I found that at the center of my experience of health was a sense of real well-being. It wasn't a muted "I feel fine" feeling. It was more like the feeling of a radiant masterpiece, something Michelangelo himself might carve. It wasn't a measurement, like my blood pressure or heart rate, nor was it the sum of many measurements. It wasn't a concept, an idea, or an emotion. The masterpiece went beyond these limited experiences, yet was always available when I turned my attention to it.

I found that giving more and more attention to that masterpiece within naturally led to lifestyle changes that improved my well-being. I saw similar masterpieces in every person I encountered—every patient, every colleague, every friend, every stranger. Health, I discovered, is a part of that masterpiece. It's a particular aspect of well-being. Immediately the thought came to me, *This has to be taught in medical school. This has to be taught in every school.*

A focus on well-being in a true <u>health care system</u> will demand a collective shift in our perspective. We must unabashedly inquire into health and well-being with the same rigor we use to attack disease. This has already begun, as is evident in the development of patient-centered care, the wellness movement, narrative medicine, mind-body medicine, and <u>integrative medicine</u>.

The sciences of psychoneuroimmunology and epigenetics—having demonstrated for decades how our well-being can be affected by the mind—are now being acknowledged by medical science. We are on the cusp of a shift in the modern understanding and achievement of health and well-being that will transform the <u>medical treatment system</u>.

You are a critical part of that shift.

A true <u>health care system</u> must be a collaboration among people representing every walk of life, an integration of its many stakeholders. Who doesn't have a stake in well-being? The time has passed for dividing health care into particular groups or specialties while ignoring the crucial need to work together.

The idea that a few key stakeholders are preventing much-needed change is incomplete and self-defeating. Every organization, including every type of health care organization, is comprised of many different kinds of people. I have found that there are some who are eager for change in even the most buttoned-down organizations. They are looking for a better way, a more fulfilling way. These change makers will be instrumental in developing a new system, each informed by his or her particular expertise.

A true <u>health care system</u> is built on inclusion, evidence, and experience, with a place for everyone—every kind of patient, practitioner, and educator. It is a system that understands and honors all aspects of the human experience, not just physical parameters. We are so used to one way of doing things—pills and procedures—that opening up the doors to include new approaches can feel threatening. Regardless, this is the future. In fact, it is the present. It is happening already.

Make no mistake, it will take a different perspective for medical institutions to unlock true health care. But, based on my conversations with patients in the ED, colleagues, friends, family, and just about anyone, there's a real readiness for a fresh perspective, a real recognition that we can't keep going in the direction we're headed in, and real empathy for the millions of patients and clinicians who are suffering. Most importantly, there is a real willingness to act anew, based on a true understanding of the nature of health and the human being. What is needed is for this international community of change makers to coalesce around that understanding.

If we want things to change, we must start at the root of the problem: How we perceive the human body and how we define <u>health</u>. We must look at ourselves in a new way, daring to ask the questions that the <u>medical treatment system</u> seems to have forgotten:

What is health?
What is well-being?
How can we experience well-being?
What is the role of a true <u>health care system</u> in fostering well-being?

Only by exploring these questions can we clearly see the nature of the distortion in the <u>medical treatment system</u> and create a new balance. This exploration must be a full, experiential one; it cannot be merely an intellectual exercise. An intellectual conversation can get us started, but by itself it will invariably end in misunderstanding because the experience of well-being is not an intellectual "fact" that can be found in textbooks.

We have all been promised solutions before. This time we have to dive in to discover them. There simply is no other way. The responsibility is ours. Don't just ask for proof. Endeavor to find it within your own experience and see how it can be applied.

The good news is that we humans are born explorers. Each of us looks for ways to live the healthiest and happiest life possible. The key is to focus the search and closely examine some of the assumptions we've held for generations about our own bodies and our health.

To bring well-being into this century, we will have to look beyond our limited vision of the nature of the body and the emphasis on the physical causes of disease. We will have to explore the connections among our Three Bodies—the Physical, the Mental, and the Energetic—three aspects of ourselves that have been described in wisdom traditions around the world for millennia. Most importantly, we will have to build a bridge between what we discover and the current <u>medical treatment system</u>.

In this book, we will show that it's time to redefine and complete our understanding of human <u>anatomy</u>. Redefining the human body in a realistic but broader way will give us the opportunity to gain knowledge and share it across disciplines. This will be the foundation on which to build a comprehensive, collaborative, true <u>health care system</u> with well-being its prime goal.

My wish is that by the end of this book you will understand yourself more completely and have the necessary knowledge to create change with your own hands. You will have a comprehensive platform from which to advocate for true health care in your own unique, valuable way. Most of all, you will discover how attending to your own well-being is the beginning of radical action.

CHAPTER 3
Two Worlds

Do something, Doc! He can't breathe!!" The patient's wife is wild-eyed. She sees her husband's chest heaving, his skin pale and clammy. He doesn't respond to her calls.

I'm zoomed in to my own body. Every cell wants to jump into action. It's what I'm trained to do. I know the textbook answer: Place a breathing tube down the patient's trachea and connect it to a ventilator so it can breathe for him. Without it, he may die any minute. It's time to act.

In the meantime, the intravenous line has already been placed. The blood samples have been collected. The nurse looks at me, her eyes saying, "What are you going to do, Doctor?" Zooming out, I review the situation in my mind.

This eighty-six-year-old gentleman has been sick for years. Numerous tests, procedures, treatments, admissions to hospitals, and visits to clinics have made him an unwilling expert on the ins and outs of medical treatment. I zoom out further. Once he goes on a ventilator, he may never come off it.

Would he want this? What does well-being mean to my patient? He never got around to having that talk with his wife. Zooming back in to the situation, I place orders with the nurse, hold his wife's hand, and begin a conversation with her.

Several hours later, I walk back to my car to head home after what feels like a very long shift. It's 3:14 a.m. on an early December morning. I turn on the heater, waiting for the cold air blowing on my feet to warm up and the frosty crystals on the windshield to melt. I think about that patient teetering between life and death. I see his wife's eyes and feel her heart pound. Well-being meant something different to each of them.

In the heat of the moment, his wife's first reaction was to do everything possible to keep him alive. But when I explained to her exactly what that meant—a breathing tube, a mechanical ventilator, and a large intravenous catheter that approached the heart—she had second thoughts. She realized that, as hard as it was for her not to exhaust every option available, her husband did not want this.

Her final decision was for us to continue to treat him medically, but defer any major procedures, such as mechanical ventilation. She felt this was the decision her husband would have made, as difficult as it was for her to make it alone. In the span of a few moments, a critically ill patient and his family had to come to terms with life, death, and everything in between.

The car warms up and I begin the drive home. My body keeps driving while my mind takes a different course home, back to my childhood...

The unmistakable aroma of freshly roasted cashews, or *parangaandi*, wafts through the air. I know instantly that my grandmother must have picked them from the cashew tree in the front yard and is grilling them in the fire. I'm four years old, playing outside in the sand in the small village of Chunnakkara in South India. I'm free. No worries.

I have thousands of toys—the leaves and stones all around me. Stones are little bits of imagination—jigsaw pieces that fit together like the chapters of a book. Each stone is unique. It comes from somewhere. It was fashioned somehow by the elements. And its destiny nobody yet knows, not even the earth beneath my feet that has witnessed the coming and going of more seasons than the oldest person in the village.

Some stones are flat and form the foundation of my fortress. It isn't the flatness of a metal sheet or of a tabletop, but the flatness of stone—a rolling, uneven flatness that seems utterly content with its apparent imperfections. And the colors! I love the ones with the brownish-orange hue. It's as if the earth and the sun had met at sunset and bled into each other, eventually cooling off and leaving behind this wondrous stone as a token of their fatal love affair.

The smaller, rounder stones make the crowning pieces. They are just round enough. Any more round and they wouldn't stay in place. They *couldn't* stay in place. Stones can be difficult, you know. Many moments are spent rotating all the pieces, finding the right angle at which they can sit.

MICHELANGELO'S MEDICINE

It's always the little crack in the stone—the deformity in an otherwise perfectly carved jewel—that allows it to maintain its perch, contributing to the whole structure. In between the foundational and crowning stones are every other shape of rock. They form the middle of the fortress, balanced on flatter stones and supporting rounder ones.

And so my imagination grew, stone by stone, structure by structure. But what holds these structures together? Ah, that is something altogether different. Whereas the stones shape the structure, the leaves make it possible. Two stones don't always sit well together. They can be hard, abrasive, and awkward. Stones are not much for conversation. Conversation is for the leaves. Supple and otherworldly, leaves make the otherwise earthbound stones buoyant.

As a child I imagined the leaves whispering their secrets to the stones, who sat silently absorbing every utterance, entranced by the green angels that mingled among them. When two stones refused to cooperate, I used a leaf as a go-between. A leaf has a way of accommodating a stone's hardness. Where a stone's surface stubbornly changes angles, leaving a gap that may destabilize the structure, the leaf glides in, effortlessly providing a supportive platform on which to build. Using some combination of the two, I built mountains.

In the ED, clinicians are sometimes stones, other times leaves. Sometimes a shortage of time can turn us to stone, and a fresh breath of air can render us a leaf. We juggle the stone and the leaf within us. Both have a role.

The <u>science</u> we learn is made from slabs of stone we call concepts. We build conceptual models of disease and treatment, stone by stone, until we develop a structure we can place our faith in during even the tensest of times. But concepts, like stones, can butt heads and become unstable. They leave gaps. Into the gaps of science, art arrives as a mediator.

In the short time that I was in India, between my third and fifth birthdays, I had the privilege of living in paradise. Sand between my toes. Plentiful trees and lush fields as far as the eye could see. More mangoes, jackfruits, papayas, bananas, and coconuts than I could possibly eat, though I tried to devour all I could get my hands on.

Our house gave us shelter, but it was less a man-made structure than an extension of the nature around us. Rain or shine, the doors were always open. The tiled clay roof overhung every entrance to the house. Even in a heavy rain, the doors could be left wide open and our home would stay dry inside.

During the monsoon season, the smell of rain and earth would permeate the rooms of the house. The rhythm of the rains would vary with each downpour, sometimes the thick, heavy, steady strike of the bass drum and at other times the shrill, rapid crescendo of the cymbal. Nature is music and music is nature, if only we listen.

I learned then that the boundary between me and the world around me was not so rigid. I felt that I didn't end at my skin, nor did I begin as a cell.

I loved the rain. I remember grabbing an umbrella and walking through the fields in the warm rain, the mud overrunning the edges of my sandals and seeping between my toes with each step. I imagined that my toes were caught in a landslide, one moment sinking perilously into the soggy, hungry earth, and in the next moment being airlifted to safety in preparation for another messy landing.

Almost everything we needed came from what was around us: the rain, sun, earth, plants, and animals. Our plates were large banana leaves. Our ladles were fashioned from other, smaller leaves. The swings we played on were made from the large branches of the coconut tree. The hard shell of the coconut served as a bowl.

For a child it was paradise, but for an adult it was hard work. My grandmother toiled from dawn to dusk. I still remember her beating our wet, soapy clothes against a large rock—our washing machine. She experienced every emotion—happiness, sadness, anger, elation, and everything in between. No matter where you are in the world, we all share the same experiences. They just dress up differently.

By nightfall, the clamor of the day would quiet to a hush. There were always two conversations going on at night—my family talking inside and the insects talking outside. I enjoyed listening to the insects. It seemed they always had something to say, or rather something to sing.

One or two insects were always buzzing around the fluorescent lights in the living room. Electricity was finicky. No matter. Flashlights and kerosene lamps gave plenty of light. The heater was the sun outside and the air conditioner was the wind that blew through the open doors and windows. When it was too hot, we'd sleep. By some standards, we would have been considered poor. But nobody told me that. Life was full. It had a rhythm, and we danced to it.

Most significantly, we were surrounded by love. Was it love? Yes, I'm sure it was love. What else could it have been? I didn't need to understand the word. I could feel the joy and warmth that filled that early child's paradise. Love was everywhere, overflowing from every corner of life. It came most clearly in the form of *ammumma*, my grandmother, who I think was an undercover agent with a not-so-secret mission of stuffing me so full of love that it would be emanating from me for all of eternity.

Those were some of the formative moments of my life. They provided a contrast to the life I would walk into when I returned to the suburbs of the United States. Even today, I look at situations through the eyes of that child to gain a new perspective, to see what else is possible.

I remember the excitement surrounding the day we returned to the United States. Being just five, I couldn't know the full significance of the move, but I did know that we would be leaving our village home, leaving the plants and animals, leaving a life that was not bounded by doors and windows, and, of course, leaving *ammumma*.

Although I was born in the United States and spent the first couple years of my life here, my first strong memory of this country came when I touched down upon returning from India. My mother, sister, and I landed at Dulles Airport on a chilly fall evening. My father had preceded us a few months earlier to start working and find us a place to live. He led us from the baggage claim to the parking lot, where a shiny, light-blue Ford Escort wagon was waiting.

Soon we were cruising down I-495, heading toward Maryland. I was allowed to ride shotgun and could barely contain my excitement. The well-paved roads, clearly marked lanes, and varieties of vehicles on the road were captivating. I practically had my nose pressed against the windshield. I had never seen lane markers before; they seemed like art to me. I wondered what more there must be to see in this amazing land that had thought to paint lines on the road! I was Alice and this new home was Wonderland.

That touching down was a significant moment. I often look back and reflect on it as the first major transition in my life. It marked the beginning of a transition from a child mind to an adult mind. I was thinking more. Questioning more. Seeking more experiences.

I was aware that something was changing, but I had neither the vocabulary to express it nor an interest in doing so. My life just seemed like a grand experiment, and I was too caught up in watching the dramatic events unfold to consider trying to talk about it.

I noticed that most adults were also seeking out new and exciting experiences, just like me. But where do we want to go? What do we really want? Deep down, what we really want—what every one of us really wants—is the experience of the masterpiece within us.

There is something stirring deep within us, calling us to remember it. It is not nostalgia for the old but the recognition of something ever-fresh, ever-new. And it holds the key to well-being.

CHAPTER 4
Is Anatomy in the Eye of the Beholder?

I remember marveling at the intricate <u>anatomy</u> of the forearm and hand in cadaver lab. It brought memories of Halloweens past when people would dress up as skeletons and extend their bony hands, asking for candy. Now I was seeing the real thing.

The forearm's array of muscles, tendons, nerves, and blood vessels captured my attention. The detail was exquisite, so much so that it was sometimes hard to believe that the body was dead. Long after the heart within that body had stopped beating, its structure was still intact. When I pulled on the tendons of the forearm, the fingers still moved. It was as if a few traces of life had wiggled in between the muscles and tendons, waiting to be activated by a curious medical student.

What struck me in particular about the human hand is its impeccable alignment of anatomy and physiology. The ropes and pulleys in the hand are perfectly formed for muscle contraction. The image that comes to mind is that of a Swiss watchmaker meticulously adjusting the components—a degree or two here, a millimeter there—so that the fingers move beautifully, even artfully. The form and function of each structure are intertwined, woven into each other. It is only conceptually that we can separate the two.

One of the courses I was taking concurrently with anatomy was histology—the study of microscopic structures. While looking through the microscope, it struck me that anatomy and histology were not two different disciplines. Add a microscope to the study of anatomy and voila—histology appears!

Another course I was taking was embryology, the study of anatomy prior to the moment the baby is delivered by the mother. I saw that using different lenses to understand the structure of the human being yielded different perspectives and different answers to the question, "What are we made of?"

While anatomy is about form, physiology is about function. Anatomy is the map while physiology is how nature navigates the terrain. Yet the two are not different. Physiology is anatomy set to music. Imagine looking at drawings and models of the heart, one at a time. This is basic anatomy. Now imagine flipping through thousands of drawings of the heart placed sequentially, each one showing the heart in successive stages of pumping blood. This is the motion picture we call physiology.

Anatomy cannot be known independently from physiology unless we press *pause* while watching the video. Freezing the frame can make anatomy deceptive because what we see depends on which frame is selected. It becomes a story without context. It turns a person into a single picture.

Anatomy and physiology are most distinct in the Physical Body. We see their clear separation when the body dies, as physiology abandons anatomy for the first time. Anatomy is never the same again. Without function, form, too, is lost. They are not that different after all. It is this form, disintegrating by the moment, that the new medical student studies.

In every cadaver of every medical school, there is hope—hope for new knowledge, hope for a cure, hope for longevity, and hope for less suffering. On the first day of anatomy lab, that hope is transferred from the cadaver to the medical student for safe keeping. There, in the depths of the sincere student's heart, hope patiently waits through stages of incubation and growth until it finally blooms as the ability to heal, to help, and to cure. This is how medical students begin their training. With hope. With anatomy. With a cadaver. Through form, they approach function.

The Physical Body has made it easy for us to differentiate form and function. But the Physical Body is just the ground for the first lesson in anatomy and physiology. When looking at the level of the mind, form and function are not as readily distinguishable. For example, thoughts and emotions are both forms *and* functions of the mind. When you are weighing a decision, the mind takes the *form* of thoughts. When you see a friend after many years, the mind takes the *form* of an emotion—joy (or perhaps a potent mix of emotions). These forms are also functions; weighing pros and cons is the *function* of thinking. Experiencing joy is the *function* of feeling.

I remember thinking about form and function after having to sit out a tennis match in the ninth grade. I had jumped up into the air, racket held high to hit an overhead slam. I had watched Pete Sampras doing this innumerable times—leaping into the air, scissor-kicking as he ascended to intercept the ball, smashing it back for a winner. For a brief second, suspended in midair, I felt like Pete. I managed to strike the ball just right, couching it for a fleeting moment in the sweet spot of my worn strings, then sending the ball hurtling back to the other side of the court. A winner! It was a combination of some skill and a heavy dose of luck, but I was thrilled by the result.

What a short-lived thrill it was. As I landed, my right ankle inverted and a sharp pain exploded in the region of the lateral malleolus—the bony prominence on the outside of the ankle. The ankle quickly began to swell. I apologized to Jose, my doubles partner, and limped off the court.

Ankle sprains are a fixture of the ED. Many people come in because of severe pain to see if they have a fracture. From the clinical perspective, the process of decision making is fairly straightforward. Once other causes of pain are ruled out, the main question is whether the fibula is fractured or not. Many times this can be determined from the clinical exam itself. For example, if the tenderness localizes to the ligaments of the ankle and the bone is not tender on examination, then it is unlikely to be a fracture, especially if the patient is able to walk.

As far as ED evaluations go, a kid with a sprained ankle being checked for a possible fracture is about as straightforward as it gets. But when I sprained my ankle back in the ninth grade, things didn't seem so simple to me. I wondered how healing happened.

My father, a biochemist and former medical school professor in India, explained the process of inflammation to me. He talked about cytokines, neutrophils, and a host of other factors that were contributing to the swelling. It sounded familiar. I had probably learned about it in science class or from one of his large textbooks that lined my bookshelf. But the story seemed incomplete.

When I thought more about how the swelling eventually started to go down, I developed more questions. How did the body know that it was time to start calling off the cytokines? What was the first step in the process? To me the whole thing seemed mysterious, yet everybody, including the textbooks, seemed to know what they were talking about.

I imagined a little factory in my ankle, constantly running, steadily producing ligaments, tendons, and bones. When new parts weren't needed, it worked on general maintenance, making sure everything was optimized. When the ankle was injured, as in the case of my sprain, the factory went into overdrive, ramping up capacity. More blood and nutrients would come in, allowing the damaged parts to be repaired and replaced.

But I couldn't answer a key question: How was the factory managing itself? My computer science class led me to an answer.

My first exposure to computer programming was a teaching language called Karel. Learning how to code felt like becoming a mad scientist. I could make something inanimate come to life. The program understood a handful of commands, like how to make an object on the screen turn to the left (simply type in "turnleft").

The problem was that Karel could *only* turn left. The programmer had to teach it how to turn right by defining a new command, "turnright." "Turnright" was defined as three sequential "turnlefts." The idea was that if I turned ninety degrees to my left three consecutive times, the net result was the same as turning right once.

I began to wonder if that was what was happening in my body. Commands were being sent out for different things to happen. When a new situation was encountered, a different command was issued, or perhaps a new series of commands were created just for that context. It's almost like typing out a long sequence of DNA, pushing play, and watching an inanimate object start to move. But it's actually even more complex than that.

Computer programming languages are composed of 1's and 0's. The patterns they make are what computer programs consist of. In the case of DNA, its programming language is built of molecules known as nucleotides, which themselves are made of atoms. I realized that I could keep tracing back this "program" to smaller and smaller parts. What programmed the DNA's 1's and 0's? Whatever was happening "onstage" was the result of something much more subtle occurring behind the scenes.

I wanted better explanations for how the human body works. As a child I had heard a lot about the mind and how it interfaced with the body. I had noticed that emotions dramatically colored my physical experiences. If I was full of anger, my experiences were not pleasant, regardless of who or what I was interacting with. On the other hand, if I was feeling ecstatic, everything looked great—even a horror movie would become a comedy. In a very real sense, I was just interacting with my mind, not an external, independent world.

I began to wonder whether mental experience was really just a "smaller" or subtler aspect of physical experience. I didn't say anything about this in high school science class though. We were learning basic anatomy, and the mind was nowhere in our textbooks.

It started coming together for me in Mrs. Schlossnagle's eleventh-grade anatomy class. We had to dissect cats, and I was not a fan. (The smell was overwhelming; even walking down the hall to the classroom was nauseating.)

At first I was interested in observing the anatomy, the distinct muscles and organs that I had previously seen only as pictures in textbooks. As we dissected smaller and smaller structures, I began thinking, "Where does it end?" We could seemingly go forever smaller, yet never cross a certain boundary of knowledge—the boundary of physical anatomy. Memorizing endless names of ever-tinier structures didn't interest me. I wanted to know what made it all work.

I found that when I paid attention to everything around me, each individual *thing* seemed separate. The sofa was separate from the carpet, which was separate from the ceiling, which was separate from the people in the room. But when I paid attention to my own mind, the objects around me and the space they occupied seemed connected with each other and with me. When my own thoughts, feelings, sensations, and subjective experiences were given the same attention usually reserved for the objects around me, the importance of the mind and its powerful role in shaping experience became apparent.

It became especially obvious to me that anatomy need not be purely a physical phenomenon. If the mind were given as much consideration as the Physical Body, then physical boundaries weren't set in stone; they were simply perceptions. By changing the mind, we could also change the perceptions of those boundaries. I saw that anatomy was simply a way of drawing boundaries—boundaries that were in the eye of the beholder.

If I could have donned a time-traveling suit at that time, I would've fast-forwarded for a quick visit to the cadaver lab in medical school to assimilate the more profound lessons I would learn about form and function. I would've seen my intuition about the mind being confirmed in the unlikeliest of places—medical school. For the time being, however, I was preparing the ground for that new understanding of anatomy that would come over a decade later.

The word *anatomy* means "to cut up," or, more simply, to divide. The arm is an anatomical structure separate from the thorax because we see a line that divides the two. The long, slender shape of the arm is clearly distinct from the boxy dimensions of the thorax. We see the division and therefore give the two parts different names, quite appropriately. As long as a majority of us agree on what we're seeing, there's no problem. But what happens when another group sees things differently? Or when an entire culture does so?

In *The Expressiveness of the Body*, Harvard professor Shigehisa Kuriyama compares centuries-old Eastern and Western representations of the human body. He writes,

> *In Hua Shou, we miss the muscular detail of the Vesalian man; and in fact Chinese doctors lacked even a specific word for "muscle." Muscularity was a peculiarly Western preoccupation. On the other hand, the tracts and points of acupuncture entirely escaped the West's anatomical vision of reality.*[1]

Different cultures have different perspectives on human anatomy because each culture has its own way of seeing and thinking. Each has its basic values, beliefs, and concepts that lead it to interpret the world through its unique point of view. Another way of saying this is that each culture molds what we perceive in a unique way. Naturally, the healing systems arising from different cultures will have different ways of viewing and thinking about anatomy.

Allopathy is based on a perspective that emphasizes physical structures. It follows that allopaths like myself see distinct physical organs and organ systems. Acupuncture is based in an ancient healing system that emphasizes the flow of energies in the body. Accordingly, acupuncturists see tracts and points. Where the mindset is different, the perceptions of the body are different, and the resulting treatment approaches are different.

The anatomy that some healing systems recognize also doubles as physiological functions, such as in Eastern traditions where the energy meridians represent the flow of energy in the body. At this level of subtle anatomy, form and function are not as distinct as they are at the physical level; they have nearly converged. They also depart together at the time of death, making it difficult for a mind tuned to physical anatomy to appreciate their existence at all.

Physical anatomy lingers for a while longer than subtle anatomy. Dissecting any number of cadavers won't yield distinct evidence of the energy known in India as *prana* or in China as *chi*. That comes only with a deep study of life itself. Gaining an appreciation of subtle anatomy requires the ability to recognize form and function together as one. This is the trademark of a synthetic mind. While the analytic mind dissects and differentiates, the synthetic mind integrates and assimilates.

Upon recognizing this, I reexamined my own body with the goal of developing a more complete and comprehensive appreciation of anatomy. First, I threw out all the traditional boundaries that I had superimposed on it. Why did my body have to end outside my skin? Wasn't that a perception, and therefore subject to interpretation? Where exactly did my body begin? Did it have to start at my head and end with my toes? Or maybe start inside and end on the outside?

So many questions, so many assumptions, so many limitations. Once I freed myself of all of these, I saw that I had a fresh canvas. I had an opportunity to redefine the body not just in terms of what one culture believed but in a universal way that reflected the relationship between the body and life itself. I didn't know it until many years later, but by allowing myself to reconsider the boundaries of human anatomy, I would give myself the opportunity to pair a deeper understanding of the human body with the experience of well-being.

Key Points

- Anatomy is a way of describing our perception of the body. Anatomy is in the eye of the beholder.
- Different cultures perceive anatomy differently, based on the way the mind is tuned.
- Different healing systems use different models of anatomy, describing the human body from unique cultural perspectives.

References

1. Kuriyama, Shigehisa. 1999. The expressiveness of the body and the divergence of Greek and Chinese medicine.

CHAPTER 5
What is Well-Being?

If you ask any physician to tell you about coronary artery disease, they will be able to give you a detailed exposition, beginning with the idea that the disease is caused by the buildup of plaque along the walls of the blood vessels that feed the heart. This buildup is due to an inflammatory condition in the wall of the blood vessel, called the endothelium. As more and more plaque builds up, the vessel narrows and, as with a clogged drain, blood flow to the heart muscle decreases, ultimately causing a myocardial infarction, a heart attack. Nearly every physician will you tell some variation of this scenario.

Now ask your physician another question: What is well-being? You will get a variety of responses. Clearly there is no single answer. You may not even get an answer. Well-being is at once both broad and personal, an experience, not a measurable quantity.

Well-being is as difficult to pin down as life itself. Neither is easy to define. Just as well-being is often interpreted against the backdrop of disease, it is hard to talk about life without mentioning death. Oddly, life and death seem to be opposites, yet they are partners. They are constantly occurring processes happening in all levels of the body.

Red blood cells have an average life span of three months and are continuously being replaced. The cells lining your gastrointestinal tract last a mere five days. But perhaps the most intriguing study of life and death is of the largest organ of your body—your skin.

The skin is broadly divided into two layers, with the epidermis on top and the dermis underneath. The epidermis is further divided into five sublayers. The two outermost layers, the stratum corneum and the stratum lucidum, are dead cells, while the deeper layers are alive and proliferating. So is your skin dead or alive? It's both, a cycle of death and rebirth.

We can apply the same thinking to the Physical Body as a whole. My Physical Body is very alive in this moment, creating words and typing them on this laptop. But by shifting my attention to the outer layers of my skin, I can also make the case that a portion of my Physical Body, like the tips of my nails and my hair, is already dead. So which am I? Living or dying?

What we generally mean by death is the tipping point when the organism as a whole stops functioning. But even that doesn't capture the whole story. Consider the patient who is apparently only physically alive, kept on a mechanical ventilator for weeks in the intensive care unit. Life is more than the sum of all the biological activity in the body. We must apply the same subtlety to understanding well-being.

The digital revolution would have us believe that it is just about ready to drop well-being into the palm of our hands, gift wrapped. For the first time, we are gaining access to reams of data not just on populations as a whole but also on each of us as individuals. The increasing use of wearable sensors and in-home monitoring means that medical care is primed for a data deluge. Every day, quintillions of bytes of data are created, perhaps much more by the time you read these words.[1]

While the medical treatment system is still adapting to harness this new trove of data, enterprising physicians are already using the latest technology to deliver customized precision care. Instead of having his or her vital signs checked during an annual physical, a person with congestive heart failure may have his or her blood pressure, heart rate, respiratory rate, and oxygen saturation monitored twice daily (or even continuously) while at home, enabling that person's physicians to detect patterns of deterioration before the patient becomes symptomatic enough to warrant a doctor's visit.

Genomics promises a different type of personalization. One of the most popular areas of molecular biology, genomics takes us beyond vital signs and other external markers of behavior by going straight to the source of molecular information—the human genome, popularly called

DNA (deoxyribonucleic acid). Housed in the nucleus of our cells, DNA contains the instructions, the "programming," for our cells to carry out. We can now access, with your consent, your personal DNA to determine which medications will work best for you, instead of relying on a one-size-fits-all approach.

As the data deluge continues, it is imperative that our attention not stray from the challenging, fundamental questions about the true meaning of health and how to achieve and maintain it. Current technological advancements are dazzling and useful for sure, but we must keep asking:

What is well-being?
What is the role of a true <u>health care system</u> in fostering well-being?
How do we cultivate and improve well-being in the long term?

In this chapter we will begin to answer the first question, and then we will explore the answers to the other questions throughout the rest of the book. Together, these questions have the potential to set a course for experiencing ourselves in a new way and for establishing a true <u>health care system</u>. We can't afford to plow headlong through the digital revolution only to raise our heads up a decade later and wonder why well-being is still eluding us. The digital revolution is a golden opportunity to get this right.

∽

Perhaps one key to decoding well-being is to examine the increasing popularity of the <u>wellness</u> movement and see what can be learned from it. In May 2012, McKinsey and Company released a report naming "wellness" the next trillion-dollar industry.[2]

Wellness has become quite the buzzword. Every hospital now has some type of wellness program (if only in name). But wellness isn't some new fad; it's been around at least since the middle of the twentieth century.

"Wellness" was born out of the need to reinvent health. For too long, popular and scientific culture has feasted on a cosmetic understanding of health, a superficial focus, primarily on the Physical Body. The proof is found on the covers of the magazines crowding grocery store checkouts, and between the covers of biology textbooks. It's what our children see and our students learn, informing an incomplete view of health and of themselves.

The result is that a tremendous knowledge vacuum has been created within our culture, which is starving for a practical, actionable understanding of health and the whole human being. Wellness and well-being have been born into this vacuum for the specific purpose of restoring meaning to health.

Wellness went from being just another word to becoming a movement in the 1950s. Dr. Halbert Dunn, chief of the National Office of Vital Statistics, wanted to define health in a new, more comprehensive way. "High-level wellness for the individual," he wrote, "is defined as an integrated method of functioning which is oriented toward maximizing the potential of which the individual is capable. It requires that the individual maintain a continuum of balance and purposeful direction within the environment where he is functioning."[3]

According to Dr. Dunn, wellness is not just about feeling good, it's growing toward your maximum potential. This growth process is described by psychologist Abraham Maslow as "self-actualization." Maslow wrote that self-actualization is the tendency of the individual "... to become actualized in what he is potentially. This tendency might be phrased as the desire to become more and more what one is, to become everything that one is capable of becoming."[4] These words may sound abstract, but they point to a real experience that we will explore in the coming chapters.

Depending on what text you reference, wellness can be defined as physical health, physical and mental health, or achievement of your maximum potential. Whereas *health* has primarily dealt with the optimal functioning of the Physical Body, *wellness* includes cultivation of the mind and other areas of life. *Well-being*, on the other hand, implies something even more comprehensive.

In 1948, the World Health Organization put its stamp on the word *well-being* when it declared that health is "a complete state of physical, mental and social well-being, and not merely the absence of disease or infirmity."[5] This is a powerful definition, but it is incomplete. Well-being doesn't just address the physical, mental, and social aspects of the human being.

The heart of well-*being* is *being*—a person's natural state. We are, after all, human *beings*. Yet, we are often caught up in *doing, thinking,* and *feeling,* rarely recognizing that we have a choice to simply *be*. There's a constant, often unexamined pressure to jump to the next item on the checklist and keep moving from activity to activity in our daily lives. At home, there's always the next meal to think about, the next soccer game, the next trip to the grocery store, the next pickup from school, and so on. At work, there's the next promotion, the next pat on the back, the next meeting. It never ends.

Yet, *being* is always available, independent of *doing, thinking,* and *feeling*. There is no prerequisite for *being*. It is always with us—not as an abstraction, but as a sense of utter ease and equanimity that is prior to *doing, thinking,* and *feeling*. *Being* can be accessed now, as you read this, no matter who you are and what your background is. It takes only a shift in attention.

Being is not a state of physical or mental health, but something more fundamental, simpler even. The problem is that we have been conditioned to think we have to go somewhere or do something to experience the freedom and joy of *being*. We're fed the message that something needs to be improved upon, something needs to be corrected, or something needs to change. (Most advertising depends on this assumption.)

Many of the stages of "acting out" that happen in the course of a human lifetime are rooted in the search for *being*—the search for something fundamental that appears to be missing from our lives. But it isn't missing, only forgotten. When the freedom of *being* is forgotten and our attention is completely diverted into the channels of *doing, thinking,* and *feeling,* we experience a subtle sense of loss and uncertainty. And then we go on a search. It may be a formal search or an informal one. We may label it a search or we may be oblivious to the searching. But search we do. We *do* things to find that fullness. We *think* and plan about how we may get there. We *feel* (or actively resist feeling) whatever comes along the way, yearning to ride the waves of the next adventure.

The outward search for that sense of ease and completion is bound to end in failure because it was never lost to begin with, only forgotten.

In those moments when we experience the failure of the search, we experience catharsis. It may be the cathartic tantrums of the toddler, the cathartic rebellion of a teenager, or the cathartic spree of a midlife crisis. After each period of catharsis, the personality settles down into another mode of searching. The toddler learns to go to school and look up to those in higher grades. The teenager eventually gets a job and starts pursuing dreams of career-building. The middle-aged person sets new career or retirement goals.

All of these behaviors can reinforce the assumption that we are missing something fundamental. Accepting this assumption creates a never-ending checklist of "critical" tasks to do. After all, we could always do better, look better, and feel better, right? How much is good enough? Certainly, actions do need to be taken in life, but they need not distract us from what has never been lost, from what is central, complete, and always available to us as human *beings*—*being* itself, the core of the masterpiece.

It is *being* that makes well-being unique and separates it from health and wellness. Health and wellness address doing, feeling, and thinking, while well-being also goes straight to your core, *being*.

In the ED, patients are often sidetracked from *being* by the catalog of diseases and medications assigned to them by the medical treatment system. On every shift I work, I see many patients who are taking more than ten medications, sometimes up to twenty or more. Many times, a prescription is for a single symptom, such as constipation, tingling in the feet, or back pain. Sometimes the medication works, but often the symptoms experienced by a patient on ten medications are the cumulative side effects of the medications themselves.

I've seen that the constant barrage of symptoms—and the worry and anxiety they cause—often are a barrier to recognizing *being*. These manifestations block out what could otherwise be the beginning of a more complete solution—one that that could begin with the patient gaining insight into why his or her symptoms may be occurring to begin with. So much attention gets focused on symptoms, medicines, and side effects that the person inside the patient, the real human being who needs attention, gets lost along the way.

The good news is that even in the face of such powerful distractions, *being* is ever-present: it is a part of us, after all. We don't have to pay extra or add it on as an option. But when it is not recognized, well-being can seem so far away, even nonexistent. This is what happens in the medical treatment system—*being* goes unrecognized, so there is no path to well-being, only disease mitigation. With nothing more substantial than disease to build on, medical science blindly grabs ahold of physical symptoms, unable to see the rest of the human being.

To bring the medical treatment system in line with the experience of well-being, each of us— including those involved in any capacity with the medical treatment system—must first learn to recognize *being*.

Here are two reflective questions that can point toward *being*:

- If I closed my eyes and suspended all my beliefs and thoughts for a few moments, what would remain?
- What is the backdrop against which I recognize my thoughts and feelings?

It is important to recognize that *being* is not the same as excitement or riding a high. Those are mental experiences that are superimposed on the state of *being*. *Being* itself is the background. It's the stage on which experiences play out. Having recognized *being*, we can cultivate the behaviors that foster well-being in all areas of life.

It can be very helpful to dedicate time to simply *be*. It can help us recognize what well-being in all areas of our life truly means—balancing all aspects of ourselves. Without that context, anything that feels good in the moment, including addictive behaviors, can be misinterpreted as well-being.

I remember a time in medical school when I was feeling pleased that I could come up with the right answers to questions from my supervising physicians. Initially, I was delighted, but when I checked in with my own sense of *being*, I recognized that I was actually feeding an addiction— one that was supported and even encouraged. While it was important to know the right answers and increase my medical knowledge, I also recognized another part of me that wanted validation from the supervising physicians.

I didn't enjoy discovering that I sometimes compromised what I thought was the right thing to do just to satisfy a need for approval.

What initially felt like delight was actually rather dull and unremarkable when I checked in with *being*. I wondered then how something as subtle and important as *being* should fit into our understanding of the human being. How did it influence the Physical Body? Where did it belong in the scheme of medical training? How could it be pointed to and recognized?

I again saw that making room for *being* meant broadening or reframing my old definitions of the human being. I resolved to learn answers for the purpose of discovering, for my patients and myself, what well-being and healing truly are, regardless of where that took me.

Surprisingly, it took me to the ED.

Key Points

- Wellness and well-being are responses to an incomplete understanding of health.
- The heart of well-being is *being*. *Being* is accessible in this very moment by anyone, regardless of external circumstances.
- We must prioritize and explore well-being to harness the full potential of the digital revolution.

Q&A

- Q: *Don't I have to eat right and do all the other things that people always talk about to be well?*
  A: Well-being is a combination of well and *being*. The *well* part of the word requires action in different areas of life, which we will further discuss in the chapter on The Four Pillars. Accessing *being* doesn't require any external action, only turning our attention inward and recognizing what has been forgotten.

References

1. http://www-01.ibm.com/software/data/bigdata/what-is-bigdata.html. Accessed 2/15/16.
2. http://www.mckinseyonmarketingandsales.com/sites/default/files/pdf/Consumer_Health_Wellness.pdf. Accessed 2/15/16.

3. H. L. Dunn, *High Level Wellness* (Thorofare, NJ: Charles B. Slack, 1977).
4. A. Maslow, *Motivation and Personality* (New York: Harper, 1954).
5. Preamble to the Constitution of the World Health Organization as adopted by the International Health Conference, New York, June 19–22, 1946.

CHAPTER 6
Angel in the ED

There I was, a newlywed and a new intern, two beginnings woven together, inaugurating my emergency medicine residency training at an inner-city hospital in the City of Brotherly Love. The work was intense. Gunshot wounds, stabbings, heart attacks, strokes, and life-threatening infections—all day, every day. It was my intention to find the needle of well-being somewhere in that blazing haystack.

When I began my internship, many of the healthy habits I had developed fell by the wayside. For example, in my last year of medical school, I had made a habit of meditating daily. That was difficult to sustain during my internship, when I wasn't getting adequate sleep. Nevertheless, I tried.

As a child I had often meditated in the conventional manner—sitting with legs crossed, closing my eyes, and focusing on my breathing. Over time, I grabbed a few minutes of meditation whenever I could. I needed that flexibility during my time-demanding internship. I found that meditating was an effective way to enhance my own appreciation of well-being alongside the disease-focused system in which I was operating. At that time I was not ready to balance and assimilate those two realities.

In my training hospital, the ED was divided into three pods: A, B, and C. The B-pod was generally staffed by only a supervising physician and, at times, one resident. It had fewer beds, and generally its patients did not have life-threatening conditions. The C-pod could handle more volume and was staffed with more residents, meaning that sicker patients could usually be expected there.

As you might expect, the A-pod was the largest patient care area, with the most beds and a designated trauma bay with three more dedicated trauma beds. The ambulance entrance fed straight into A-pod. It was the place where anything could happen at any time.

As residents, we were like the infantry, manning the trenches in the battle against disease. It didn't have to be coronary artery disease, bowel obstructions, splenic lacerations, or respiratory failure, it was *dis-ease* itself that we fought. Patients came to the ED because they were uneasy. Something was wrong.

Deep down, I recognized that well-being was always present in my patients in some form, often buried under layers of disease. I knew this, but I had a very difficult time unearthing it for my patients and myself. Usually, my task was to find the weed of disease and pull it out, if not by the root then at least by whatever symptom surfaced above ground. Well-being was an afterthought, usually not even that.

Residency is a time when young physicians hone their clinical skills under the supervision of experienced physicians. Having been tied to books and exams for the better part of four years, we are now able to apply what we've learned in the real world of patient care.

When I started my residency in emergency medicine, we were still using handwritten note sheets to document clinical encounters. Every note began with the *chief complaint*, the reason the patient had come to the ED. It was often the first thing a patient said. "My stomach hurts," or "I had a seizure," or "I don't feel good."

In most cases the chief complaint is presented on a platter (assuming the patient is awake and can speak), but that platter can also mislead. For example, the chief complaint of *abdominal pain* may end up having little to do with any of the organs in the abdomen.

Patients often pause after the chief complaint. That's what Mrs. Benini did when I saw her in my first year of residency. She volunteered that her stomach was hurting, but then kept quiet. I tried to do what all good physicians are supposed to do and wait for her to continue. Nothing.

Within seconds, I became impatient. I was hungry, I had to use the restroom, I hadn't slept well in days, I had other patients to see (to meet my unofficial quota and be a productive resident), and above all, the ED was unforgivingly loud. To say the least, I was very distracted, and after a few meager moments of attempted silence, I couldn't bear it. I had to dive in. I had to *keep going*. I tried asking Mrs. Benini open-ended questions.

"Can you tell me more about that?"

"It just hurts," she responded.

I could feel my impatience growing, along with my sense of inadequacy and self-judgment. *Where were the benefits of meditation when I needed them? Was I shrinking in my white coat? Would Mrs. Benini notice? She must know I'm an intern. She'll probably ask for a real doctor any moment now.*

Frustrated, not sure what else to do, I barreled forward with specifics, even though I judged I should've waited longer. Waiting always yields information. Even silence is information. But I convinced myself that I had no time and there were other patients to see.

Where does it hurt? I was narrowing down the possible organ systems involved.

When did it start? I was trying to re-create a scenario in my mind.

What were you doing when it started? She gave me a quizzical expression.

Have you had this same pain before? I was trying to give context to her symptoms.

As I ran through the standard list of questions, I realized that I was boxing Mrs. Benini in. This wasn't the open-ended conversation I was supposed to be having. I was defining her condition for her, "asking" her to describe what happened in a way that made it easy for me to treat her, not in a way that told me how she actually experienced her symptoms.

If she told me about her experience in her own words, would I understand? That was a scary thought. I was a physician. I was supposed to understand. But every patient is different. Two people with the exact same diagnosis often tell very different stories. I've had many patients who didn't see the point in localizing their discomfort, meaning that even if their physical exam suggested that the pain was in their upper abdomen, they wouldn't say more than a simple, "It hurts" when asked where their pain was located.

Does the pain radiate anywhere?

Is it worse if you eat or drink something?

Like a racehorse with blinders on, I had only one path forward. Asking pointed questions, I began to steer the story in a direction I was more comfortable with. I was not really doing anything *wrong*, per se. In fact, I was pretty much going by the book. But I couldn't help but wonder what she would say if I allowed her to tell it her way. What hidden problems might she reveal?

And this was for a stomachache. What about the patient with a subtle stroke? The patient with a small blood clot in the lung, causing her to feel ever so slightly uneasy? Would I pick up on their *dis-ease?* Disease, it seemed to me, could be identified only when it stood apart from the background of well-being, and it was difficult to get a sense for the patient's experience of well-being without letting the patient talk about it in his or her own words.

If I didn't know what well-being was—if I hadn't studied it, experienced it, shared it, and essentially immersed myself in it—how could I really know about its lack, which is disease? And how would I ever pick up on the subtleties of disease? What if it were possible to detect disease before it became a chief complaint, before the patient could give voice to it? Would I ever know? Would medical care ever know?

I had many more questions than answers. I was unable to unquestioningly go along with what I viewed as a limited understanding of medicine being applied to patients who were much too multifaceted, lively, and filled with personality to be contained by it.

> "The scientific world-picture vouchsafes a very complete understanding of all that happens — it makes it just a little too understandable. It allows you to imagine the total display as that of a mechanical clockwork which, for all that science knows, could go on just the same as it does, without there being consciousness, will, endeavor, pain and delight and responsibility connected with it — though they actually are. And the reason for this disconcerting situation is just this: that for the purpose of constructing the picture of the external world, we have used the greatly simplifying device of cutting our own personality out..."[1]
> — ERWIN SCHRODINGER, NOBEL PRIZE–WINNING PHYSICIST

I wished I could shrug it off. After all, we were working our tails off. I recognized the importance of the service we were providing by stabilizing patients, alleviating pain, and managing disease. But there was still something big missing.

I asked myself over and over, what does real health, and its partner, well-being, mean in the context of medical treatment? I knew intuitively what well-being was, but didn't have anything from my medical education to correlate it with. The closest I could come up with was that we were instructed about how important it is to build rapport with our patients. Certainly, building rapport contributes to a sense of well-being in both the patient and the clinician. But my sense was that well-being reached further than that.

In medical school, I had spent so much time studying disease and treatment—pathology, pathophysiology, clinical diagnosis, pharmacology—and none at all on well-being. The days of studying how the body worked—anatomy, physiology, histology, and embryology—were still vivid in my memory, but once we had grasped those basic concepts, we moved on to disease and never looked back. We never really explored true health or well-being, doing little more than learn to address symptoms.

On my drive to work one morning, after a thirteen-hour stint in the ED the previous night, I had a flashback to anatomy lab in medical school, followed by a memory of the time I sprained my ankle in high school. Anatomy... anatomy... something about anatomy was bugging me. Then it clicked.

I couldn't put well-being and medical treatment together because my mind was stuck in a physical model of the body. That physical model alone couldn't accommodate well-being, which was much more comprehensive and nuanced than a physical system. Trying to force-fit the two together was causing me no end of grief.

I realized that I had been avoiding the unavoidable: the need to redefine and complete the version of human anatomy I was taught. Now it seemed obvious and inevitable. Bringing well-being to the <u>medical treatment system</u> would require a new take on the nature of the human body.

These were the thoughts that often accompanied me as I walked into the ED for a shift. Shift change on a busy evening in a high-acuity emergency medicine residency program is something to behold. Every room is full. Patients in stretchers line the hallways. Many more are in the waiting room and at the ambulance entrance.

The ED on a busy evening is like a gigantic balloon. The influx of patients always seems to outpace the efflux, and the balloon grows ever larger. Every new emergency is like an additional puff of air, with the balloon getting ready to blow. You're sure it's going to pop. You can even imagine the deafening sound. Only it doesn't pop ... usually. Somehow, the ED seems to defy the laws of physics, stretching thin to give you more space, shrinking back to give you more time.

Every ED doc, every nurse, and surely many patients have thought, "Is this safe? Is this good care?" The ED is designed to hold only so many people, but when your place of work and job title both have the word *emergency* in them, all limits must be flexible. Walls, physical or otherwise, can't dictate what needs to happen when there is an emergency. The seams come close to bursting but the balloon *can't* pop. There is no Plan B after the ED.

On such evenings in the ED, music is constantly blasting. No, not that kind of music. Machine music. The beeps and rings of every medical device you can imagine.

The musical singsong of a ventilator. Beep beep beep . . . BEEP BEEP! Beep beep beep . . . BEEP BEEP!

The rapid fire of a cardiac monitor. Beepbeepbeepbeep.

The ring of a patient requesting assistance. *Ding!*

But beeps and rings are just two items on the audible menu. There are also whirrs, shouts, cries, laughs, whispers, whooshes, chimes, clicks, splashes, sirens, and thuds. Questions about patient care are called out to you between the phone calls that never stop. EKGs are held directly in front of your eyes for you to sign. Once in a while the emergency phone also blares—even within the ED there are regular phone calls and emergency phone calls announcing the imminent arrival of a critically ill patient. Welcome to A-pod.

Amidst all this, your team of six huddles, going over the salient aspects of the evaluation for each of the thirty patients in the ED. *Sign out*, as the whole process is called, is coordinated chaos. As events develop, members of the team may peel off and return later. At the end of the process, it's as if we all yell "Break!" and scurry off in different directions to manage whatever needs to be done.

It was in this hectic setting on a Monday evening that I saw an elderly lady who had come to the ED with chest pain. I walked into the room and pulled the curtain closed behind me. "Hi. I'm Dr. Kumar," I said, not quite sure that I knew enough to properly make use of that title.

My white coat was still gleaming, not because it had come from the cleaners but because it had hardly been used. Here was a lady of eighty-plus years coming to seek health advice from someone who hadn't yet completed his third decade of life. I wondered how I could possibly help her. More than likely, she would be teaching me.

As I stood there, such thoughts rose up, then drifted away. A few moments later, I found that we were looking at each other in silence. The silence was so pronounced that I felt like I could actually hear it. It should've been an awkward moment, but it wasn't. It seemed perfectly natural, as if this were like every other patient encounter.

Then a most unexpected thing happened. She slowly raised her head up from the bed and looked at me more closely, then took my hand. I was holding a clipboard and a pen to document the history and physical exam. She grasped the hand with the pen in it. This was at once unexpected, and yet completely natural. There was no awkwardness. Everything was as it should've been. Holding my hand, she said, "*You are so loving.*"

There was nothing for me to say. Nothing I could say. This was not a statement to which I was able to respond. My mind was blank, still, serene—a serenity that swallowed the chaos of the ED whole. In that moment, she was right. I *felt* loving. I *felt* loved.

I was taken back to my childhood in that vibrant village in south India. I felt possibility, joy, and utter peace. In that moment, I knew what true health care could really be. We remained that way for I don't know how long. Then everything faded to white.

I don't remember anything more from that night in the ED. I don't remember that wonderful lady's name, her history or physical exam, her diagnosis, or her treatment plan. I don't remember if what she had was life threatening or not. I don't remember if she was admitted to the hospital or went home. But I do know that wherever she is, she's okay. She was like an angel who showed up in the most unexpected of ways during a crucial part of my life, reminding me of what is possible, for which I will always be grateful. She offered me a glimpse into the heart of well-being by pulling back the curtain on the masterpiece within each one of us.

I experienced healing that night. It wasn't the healing of a physical disease but of a *dis-ease* that I had been carrying with me—the anxiety of reconciling my medical knowledge with my own experience of life. I saw that all healing begins in the heart of well-being, where possibility lives.

The fingertip laceration that heals does so because the body accesses its innate wisdom—a wisdom that the rational brain cannot completely understand. That wisdom guides the repair process so precisely that even the unique friction ridges atop the outermost layer of skin are exactly reproduced as though they were the original. I saw that by accessing this innate wisdom, the body could heal itself better and in unexpected ways. I saw that our experiences of health, well-being, disease, and cure could be transformed with this wisdom. I understood that this inner dimension of *being* was as critical a component of human anatomy as any physical structure.

I also saw that the heart of well-being is not reached by *doing* anything in particular. In fact, it's the opposite. It's an *un*-doing. What is it like to just *be*? My patient that night showed me that to just *be* is to go beyond ideas, concepts, and interpretations. It is to go beyond demands, expectations, and judgments. It is to return to your core. That core *being* is unfettered by disease, pain, and suffering. It is a glimpse beyond all these to the masterpiece that is the human *being*. This is where healing begins.

Key Points

- The heart of well-being—*being*—is accessible everywhere, all the time, under any circumstances.
- *Being* is a domain of natural intelligence and possibility. This possibility includes the experience of healing.

References

1. Schrödinger, Erwin (1951). Nature and the Greeks. Cambridge University Press.

CHAPTER 7
What are the Three Bodies?

My early attempts at figuring out how to bring well-being to the <u>medical treatment system</u> included staying awake at 3:00 a.m. in the hospital's call room and sketching out what I then called "unified health," hoping my pager wouldn't go off yet again. Unfortunately, it generally would.

I'd put down my pen and paper, answer the page, and usually leave the room to go check on a patient. Sometimes it would take just a minute or two, other times an hour or more if the situation was critical. Ultimately, I'd return to the call room and again pick up the pen and paper.

I sensed the contradiction in what I was doing. On the one hand, I was trying to figure out what well-being is, while, on the other hand, I was probably compromising my own health by not sleeping whenever I had the chance, even for a few minutes. Yet, thinking about unified health gave me satisfaction—that had to count for something. I couldn't quite reconcile it all, which motivated me even more.

I remember sketching a stick figure and writing down next to it the most important ingredients of life: oxygen, water, glucose, and so on. I traced the path of each through the body. Oxygen enters the nose and mouth, then passes down through the trachea into small sacs called alveoli in the lungs. There, oxygen diffuses across a membrane and binds to the hemoglobin component of a red blood cell. The red blood cell is like the ultimate roller coaster. It zings through arteries and capillaries until it reaches the tissue that needs its passenger the most. There, it drops off oxygen and heads back to the lungs, ready to thrill the next customer.

Oxygen, meanwhile, gets ready for the big show. It makes its way to the mitochondria, which is the body's energy production center. There it does what it was born to do: catch an electron. This may sound anticlimactic, but oxygen swallowing up electrons is an important step in allowing the body to continue producing adenosine triphosphate, or ATP—the main energy molecule in the body. This is why oxygen is so important to us. It helps harness energy for when we need it. The very process of catching that electron also converts oxygen into H_2O, or water—the end of the journey.

I repeated the process of tracing the path of each ingredient many times, trying to see where the paths converged and diverged. Each time I hit the same wall that had stopped me so many times before. As important as oxygen and glucose were to life, experiences such as joy, sadness, and a sense of meaning were important as well.

I found it impossible to reduce those experiences into molecules and fit them into my diagram. Where were they supposed to go? Where did they fit into the anatomy of the human body? In a tiny neuron? How did the physical integrate the mental, or vice versa? It seemed the experiences that meant the most had no place to go. Then my pager would go off again.

I found myself thinking more and more about anatomy. I returned to an imperfect metaphor—anatomy as the body and physiology as the mind; anatomy as form and physiology as function. I recalled how crystal-clear my understanding of anatomy was in medical school; how I pored over every aspect of the human body while doing a detailed physical exam. Sometimes, a detailed exam of a patient would take up to an hour or more. Even if the patient's chief complaint was ear pain, I would examine him head to toe, even between the toes, performing a full anatomical exam. I couldn't afford to miss a single clue that might reveal the underlying physiological problem.

When Mr. Halpern came in complaining of shaking chills and ear pain, I found evidence of an infection between the first and second toes of his left foot. How were the ear pain and the toe infection related? Every medical student knows that recurrent infections, especially in the feet, raise a red flag, suggesting that the body may not be managing glucose levels properly.

In this case, Mr. Halpern's body had difficulty transporting glucose into the cells that needed it the most, a condition technically known as type 2 diabetes mellitus. His diabetes was uncontrolled, causing numbness in the feet that made it difficult for him to feel the pain of the small cut he had sustained. Untended to, the cut became infected. If the infection were to go untreated, it could rapidly spread to the point that the toe or even the lower leg would need to be amputated.

The same uncontrolled diabetes made him susceptible to infections elsewhere. When I inspected his ear, I saw that the soft cartilage of the pinna (the outside of the ear) was not flat against the side of his head, as one would typically expect, but rather protruding outward. The mastoid bone immediately behind the pinna was also exquisitely tender. This was a classic presentation of mastoiditis, an aggressive infection of the mastoid bone that was especially concerning in diabetics.

The anatomical exam of the foot and ear led me to the pathophysiology of diabetes. I had retraced the footsteps of the body from the physical to the physiological, or, as I thought of it, from the solid to the subtle. I felt that I could take it one step further. I hypothesized that if I could observe a patient carefully enough, taking note of his or her personality, lifestyle habits, gestures, and assumptions about health and disease, these observations might lead me to more fundamental information about what was initiating disease at the physiological and, ultimately, the anatomical level.

I began to see the body as a flowing process rather than a fixed structure. That process had multiple layers, each one informing the next, from subtle to sum total, until the outermost layer—the Physical Body—showed itself as the expression of multiple subtler processes. Seeing the body in this light finally gave me a place to chart experiences such as joy and a sense of meaning. These were the finer mental processes that appeared as the physical processes.

Thinking along these lines taught me that each bit of anatomy had a profound story to tell, if I had the time and inclination to listen. By looking at a worn knee, I could see the story of arthritis. I could envision the physiology of the femur and tibia rubbing against each other with minimal cartilage in between. I could see form and function not as separate elements but a single continuity. I could see the long hours the patient was spending on his feet and the pain he suffered at the end of the day. And I could see the sadness that came with the pain, since he was unable to do some of the activities that were meaningful to him.

Each of these was an ingredient of his present condition, and any of them could be acted upon to begin a change. Physical anatomy can affect the deeper layers of the human being, but it is equally true that the deeper layers can inform the physical. The story writes itself both ways.

Eventually, I would no longer have the time to complete an hour-long physical exam. As an ED doc, I had to develop the skill to zero in on key anatomical and physiological findings within seconds, or minutes at the most. Go too fast and I might miss something. Go too slow and the patient waiting in the next room would destabilize.

To complete a focused exam, I learned to make a general assessment of the patient as a whole, then tie that together with a particular organ system or area of the body. This approach quickly links the overall clinical scenario with a potential source of the problem. But an organ system does not function independently; it depends on other organ systems.

For example, the circulatory system, including the heart and the blood vessels, is the system that delivers nutrients to all of the organs, including the heart itself. But it is dependent on the lungs to replenish the oxygen in the blood so the heart receives enough energy to keep beating. The heart and lungs, in turn, depend on the liver and kidneys to filter out toxins. There is an exquisite interdependency and balance among the anatomical and physiological systems in the body. To isolate one organ system from another is to divide what is a complete unitary system.

What are the boundaries of this unitary system?

You could say that the body begins at the cellular level. A cell functions as a unitary organism. It exhibits the same functions you and I do. It drinks, eats, excretes, moves, and reproduces. It interacts with the environment around it. And it works in a community of other cells.

But zoom in to the cell and you will discover organelles, or mini organs. Zoom in further and you reach the atomic world, each atom being its own unit. Beyond that is the subatomic world of unitary particles.

Each time you zoom in, you find another building block. Once you go beyond the tiniest elements of matter that we know, elementary particles, you enter the world of energy and information, where solidity disappears into a cloud of probability. So take a guess. Where does the body begin? Where does it end?

Taking the opposite approach, if we zoom out from the cell, we see organs, also unitary structures. The liver, for example, takes in blood, excretes toxins, and regenerates tissue as needed. It works within a community of organs. If we further zoom out to the level of the human organism, again we have the same picture. But why stop there?

Consider how much we have in common with our immediate environment. When we breathe in air from the environment, it literally becomes part of us. Oxygen from the environment diffuses into our bloodstream from the lungs and circulates to all the tissues in the body. In a similar manner, the carbon dioxide we exhale becomes part of the external environment.

Light from the environment is also assimilated into the body: photons enter our eyes and are absorbed by the cells of the retina. The food in the environment literally becomes our physical bodies once we ingest, digest, and assimilate it.

At the end of our lives, our physical bodies eventually decompose into the ground, to be recycled as nutrients for the next wave of life. The Physical Body is a process that is constantly in conversation with its environment, exchanging parts and information. If we look at this plainly, it becomes obvious that we are not separate from our physical environments. Our physical environments are a very real extension of ourselves, an extended Physical Body.

In fact, we don't just have one body. We have three. But you won't find them in *Gray's Anatomy*. We don't talk about <u>The Three Bodies</u> in hospitals, clinics, or conferences because we're not trained to recognize them. Medical science has primarily mapped the Physical Body, and therefore it inevitably squeezes everyone into a physical anatomical model. We will have to practice seeing the whole person—all Three Bodies—to create a true <u>health care system</u>.

The human being is a whole organism. All boundaries drawn within that wholeness, physical or otherwise, are testaments to the way we have been trained to see it, either through formal teaching or through our very biology. Here, I present a model of the complete human being interpreted through Three Bodies. The basis for modeling the human being through Three Bodies (as opposed to greater or fewer) is that each of <u>The Three Bodies</u> is distinct and can be experienced by anyone, as we will see. Just as each of us can appreciate physical anatomy, with practice we can appreciate each of <u>The Three Bodies</u>.

This model also provides the right amount of information for it to serve as a common framework for every type of health practitioner. Since a true <u>health care system</u> will integrate the many <u>healing systems</u> of the world, there is now a need for a common vision of human anatomy to emerge so that we may start communicating across different disciplines and traditions. If the new model includes too little information, the different <u>healing systems</u> cannot be reconciled. If it includes too much information, the model will be overwhelming and unusable. <u>The Three Bodies</u> strike a balance.

What Are the Three Bodies?

(1) THE PHYSICAL BODY – The Physical Body needs little introduction; it is the body with which we are most familiar. It is the body according to medical science; the body presented in Henry Gray's textbook; the body depicted by the great medical artist Dr. Frank Netter, with whose images every medical intern in the country is familiar. This is the body enshrined by Michelangelo as David in the city at the heart of the Renaissance, Florence; the body so meticulously corrected and detailed by Leonardo da Vinci in his geometric representation of Vitruvian Man.

The Physical Body includes cells, tissues, organs, organ systems, and the organism as a physical whole. Yet, it is also more than all of these parts. The Physical Body is personal. It is the body we clothe, feed, and decorate; the body we groom, reshape, and resize; the body we seek to preserve and hope to make younger even as it ages. The personal Physical Body is the one that we have grown accustomed to recognizing.

But the Physical Body is not only the *personal* one made of flesh and blood. We also have an *extended* Physical Body. This is the environment around us, detected by our five senses of sight, hearing, smell, taste, and touch. The extended Physical Body is the extension of us in which we play, work, and live. It includes the people, places, and objects around us right now.

Why do I call the environment around us our extended Physical Body? Consider that every atom that comprises your personal Physical Body has come from the extended Physical Body around you. These atoms were formed billions of years ago after the Big Bang. They formed galaxies, our planet, our immediate environments, the food we eat, and ultimately, your personal Physical Body. In other words, your personal Physical Body is literally a recycled version of your extended Physical Body. The two are not fundamentally different.

This connection between the personal and extended Physical Bodies has direct, practical implications for well-being. If the extended Physical Body is toxic due to environmental factors or other imbalances, the personal Physical Body is likely to reflect that. Examples include pollutants in the air triggering asthma or low-quality food causing inflammatory conditions and diabetes. Such health factors (often categorized as environmental or social determinants of health) are hinting that we should reconsider whether our physical bodies truly end at the edges of our skin.

Public health experts have recognized and addressed this connection between the *extended* Physical Body and the *personal* Physical Body for a long time, although they don't use the same terminology. Clinical medicine needs to catch up. It should recognize that our Physical Body *is* the body of the environment, reorganized.

(2) THE MENTAL BODY – While the Physical Body has been enshrined by sculptors and painters, the Mental Body has been immortalized by poets and philosophers.

> *"All things are ready, if our minds be so."*
> –WILLIAM SHAKESPEARE, *HENRY V*

> *"When the mind manifests, everything else manifests."*
> –SHANKARA

The Mental Body is the internal environment comprised of the experiences of the mind. If you close your eyes and pay attention to the Mental Body, four kinds of experiences can arise: Sensations, Images, Feelings, and Thoughts. Psychiatrist Dan Siegel came up with the acronym SIFT as a convenient way to remember these four components of the Mental Body.

Other mental experiences are either combinations or more subtle forms of these four basic ones. Memories, for example, can have any or all of the four components in one package. If you recall a memory from an enjoyable birthday party, you may see an image of your friends, feel happiness, and have the thought, "That was really fun."

Our sense of identity is also in the Mental Body. For example, "I am Anoop" or "I am (your name)" is a silent thought that may constantly run in the background of the mind, often below the surface of awareness. That thought essentially defines a human being as a particular personality and Physical Body, focusing my experience through that perspective. The expression "Put yourself in his shoes" is a reminder to examine and step out of that silent assumption and experience different perspectives.

More than the Physical Body, it is the Mental Body that determines our quality of life. This is why people who are physically fit can still be stressed out and unhappy, while another person who may find it difficult to even walk can still be worry-free and fulfilled. A racing mind struggling to check every box on a long to-do list reflects the experience of stress. A calm mind with few distracting thoughts reflects the experience of contentment and joy.

An easy way to bring the Mental Body into focus is to close your eyes. The eyes bring in so much data from the external world that switching off the sense of sight can cause a dramatic shift into the Mental Body. Immediately, you are likely to become aware of a flurry of thoughts and emotions.

Sometimes this rush of mental activity can be unpleasant because these thoughts and emotions are often the ones that have been drowned out by engaging in the physical world. But this is precisely the power of the Mental Body. By attending to it, not only will you discover what your subconscious drivers have been but you can defuse them. Behavioral changes then follow naturally, releasing old habits and harnessing newly available mental resources for whichever activity you choose. On the other hand, trying to change behavior without addressing these root causes is a constant struggle that yields temporary results at best.

Take the example of Lucy, a thirty-something struggling to lose weight. For some six years she had tried every diet in the book and even joined a Zumba class. But no matter how much weight she lost (as many as fifteen pounds at a time), she would eventually gain it all back, sometimes rebounding to a heavier baseline.

Understandably frustrated and running out of options, Lucy decided to try meditation. For the first few weeks she dedicated just ten minutes a day to the practice, and in the beginning it was just another frustrating experience. Her thoughts would race. Her emotions were overwhelming. She would vividly recall arguments she thought she'd forgotten. She considered quitting, but realized that going back to the same old seesaw dieting routine would make her miserable, so she stuck with it.

Gradually, with just ten minutes of daily meditation, Lucy began to feel lighter, less burdened. She couldn't exactly figure out how or why. She still had strong food cravings and would sometimes still binge, but she stopped beating herself up over it. Lucy's Mental Body was clearing itself out and becoming more efficient.

Lucy appreciated the change in her quality of life so much that she increased her practice to twenty minutes twice a day. She found that her craving to overeat further diminished. She was more excited about making her Zumba classes regularly. Soon her binges were exceptions rather than regular behavior. She no longer had to make losing weight her primary focus. The subconscious drivers of her behavior changed enough that her Physical Body reflected them by naturally shedding a few pounds.

As Lucy discovered, experiencing the Mental Body does not mean we must have our eyes closed. This is a common misinterpretation. Most of our time is already spent inhabiting the Mental Body. Closing the eyes is just a way of starting to recognize it. Let's take an example to illustrate this point.

Imagine that a person who could barely afford to pay his rent and was on the verge of eviction just got a large, unexpected raise. He is likely to feel exhilaration. The emotion he experiences is overwhelming.

If he gets up to walk in his emotionally overwhelmed state, he may even stumble over something. Even though his eyes are open and his Physical Body is moving around, he is still primarily experiencing the Mental Body because his attention is primarily on his own thoughts and emotions.

If you examine your own experience in this moment, you will see that you are likely inhabiting the Mental Body. As you read these words, you are interpreting their meaning and significance through thinking. This is the Mental Body.

These examples reveal an interesting conclusion. Even though we are apparently interacting with a physical world at the level of the Physical Body, it is really our minds that are interfacing with the world. We are gathering data through our eyes, ears, nose, tongue, and skin, synthesizing it, forming an interpretation, and then responding.

Although the Mental Body is quite real experientially, we traditionally don't think about it as a body. This is simply a convention of language. The Mental Body grows and develops just as the Physical Body does. It is as real an experience as the Physical Body. But because science and popular culture have given so much importance to the personal Physical Body, they have not yet recognized the full significance of the broader, powerful Mental Body.

Lucy's weight loss is an example of how just how powerful and real the Mental Body is. It demonstrates that what we call the Physical Body can be seen as a crystallized form of the Mental Body. Lucy found that as her Mental Body changed, her Physical Body automatically reflected that change. There was no distinct boundary between them.

(3) THE ENERGETIC BODY – If the Physical Body inspires sculptors and the Mental Body inspires poets, the Energetic Body inspires adventurers.

The Energetic Body is the subtlest of <u>The Three Bodies</u>. Nobody disputes the existence of the Physical Body. We can all see and touch it. Few would dispute the existence of the Mental Body, although some might call it by a different name. (After all, we can all recognize that we have thoughts and feelings that drive us to action.)

The Energetic Body is different. It is subtle enough that it can easily go unnoticed by a mind sustaining a constant flow of thoughts and emotions, just as a boulder at the bottom of a river can remain unnoticed as long as the water at the surface is turbulent. Turbulence is relative in this example. Even a steady flow of unexamined thought can mask the Energetic Body. This is why the Energetic Body is unknown to science today. Popular science is the process of using the mind to look outward. It does not endeavor to still the mind and look inward beyond its own assumptions, which is where the Energetic Body lives.

Being the subtlest of <u>The Three Bodies</u>, the Energetic Body is also the most powerful. Just as the Mental Body influences our Physical Body through emotions and thoughts, the Energetic Body influences even the deepest layers of the Mental Body—what we may call the subconscious or latent mind.

Exploring and operating from the Energetic Body can create dramatic changes. Previously, we saw that Lucy noticed differences in her life after she began meditating. As Lucy continued cultivating a meditative state, over time she began to experience ever-deeper layers of her Mental Body, ultimately reaching her Energetic Body. While exploring her Energetic Body, she experienced changes in her relationships, changes in her career, and, much to her delight, a healthier weight that remains stable. (Notably, it wasn't the weight she had initially set her sights on.) It wasn't easy, but ultimately Lucy was happy with the result. Such dramatic changes are often labeled *transformative* because so many aspects of life evolve that the individual is seemingly transformed into a new version of him- or herself.

For some, the Energetic Body can seem imaginary, abstract, or out of reach. It is only natural for it to seem so. Given the limitations of what we are taught about the human body from elementary school through medical school, it is common for our Mental Bodies to harbor a host of assumptions that make a deeper understanding of human anatomy difficult, even though this knowledge has existed in other cultures for millennia.

Yoga and traditional Chinese medicine, for example, have interpreted and mapped the Energetic Body in exquisite detail. But because energetic anatomy is not visible to the naked physical eye, these maps have not been understood by science. Studying a map is not the same as navigating the terrain, after all. In this case, navigating the terrain requires dedicating time for the journey.

The Energetic Body is often recognized for the first time when the Mental Body has quieted to a hush. It shows its first traces differently in each person and easily can be overlooked at first. You may notice it as a new feeling of heat or warmth spreading through the body. You may notice a buzzing sensation within the body, or an involuntary change in your breathing pattern and posture. You may experience the sudden release of emotions, ones you didn't know were there.

These sensations are easy to overlook and dismiss because they can be interpreted as being only mental or physical. (Indeed, in the beginning they may be so.) The key is to remain aware of these sensations as they arise while letting go of the mental tendency to hang on to them. This will allow mental turbulence to eventually subside, clearing the view to the Energetic Body.

Connecting with the Energetic Body can feel like being hooked up to a battery and getting charged. As you continue charging, you may experience what feels like a current flowing throughout your Mental and Physical Bodies. You won't have to imagine this flow; you will experience it. Other experiences may accompany this—some profound, some unremarkable. Each person's experience is unique. The more ideas we superimpose on what the Energetic Body is or should be, the greater the mental turbulence and the less the Energetic Body shows itself.

The best thing about the Energetic Body is that it doesn't require any belief, only a spirit of adventure. All Three Bodies can be recognized through established <u>introspective methods</u>, such as reflection and meditation. If you wish to recognize and experience your Three Bodies, start by taking the time to explore yourself.

Our Three Bodies are interconnected. We are as much a part of each other and of the environment as we are unique organisms. <u>The Three Bodies</u> operate in unison, freely interfacing with and informing each other. A change in one body suggests that change is occurring in the other two as well, even if it is unrecognized.

Let's say you've wanted to learn how to paint since you were a child. For whatever reason, this always got pushed to the back burner. Now, at age forty-five, you've decided you're finally going to go for it. That movement toward painting is occurring simultaneously in all Three Bodies.

Your Energetic Body activates your Mental Body and makes you aware of the desire to paint, which, in turn, prompts your Physical Body to sign up for a painting class and start putting paintbrush to canvas.

A person who is unaware of the Energetic and Mental Bodies won't recognize the mechanics of how this happens, but it happens nonetheless. A person who is aware of the Mental Body might say, "All I can think of is painting. I even dream about it." A person who is aware of the Energetic Body may or may not say anything, but will move with ease to direct that energy toward making painting a reality.

Another example of the interconnectedness of The Three Bodies is how mental activity creates physiological changes in the Physical Body. Anger and anxiety are both experienced in the Mental Body, but they also have a characteristic energy associated with them from the Energetic Body. Anger is an intense energy, which is why suppressed anger can cause mental and physical imbalances. Both anger and anxiety generally cause changes in the Physical Body, including increases in blood pressure, heart rate, and respiratory rate and dilation of the pupils. Addressing anger and anxiety in the Mental Body can be helpful, while addressing it in the Energetic Body can be transformative.

Thus, the Energetic Body fuels the Mental Body, which, in turn, molds the personal Physical Body from the materials of the extended Physical Body. Each body can be thought of as one unit of the whole human organism. It is equally correct to see the whole human organism as one unit, comprised of each of The Three Bodies. This is just like saying that the heart is one unit and the blood vessels are a separate unit, while also seeing that the cardiovascular system is a whole unit unto itself, comprised of both the heart and the blood vessels.

The concept of *my body* is an incomplete story. You and I do not begin with the atoms comprising our cells, nor do we end at the external surface of our skin. Right now, our Mental Bodies are interfacing through these words. We share an extended Physical Body. Where do my bodies end and yours begin?

We cannot draw arbitrary lines in human anatomy like we do on maps. Classical physical anatomy is *one* way of dividing the body up, but not the only way. Restricting the cultivation of well-being to only the Physical Body, or even to only the Physical and Mental Bodies, simply will not do anymore. You are much more than your Physical Body. You are *being* itself, expressing through Three Bodies and functioning seamlessly as a unitary organism. This understanding and experience is central to bringing well-being within our reach.

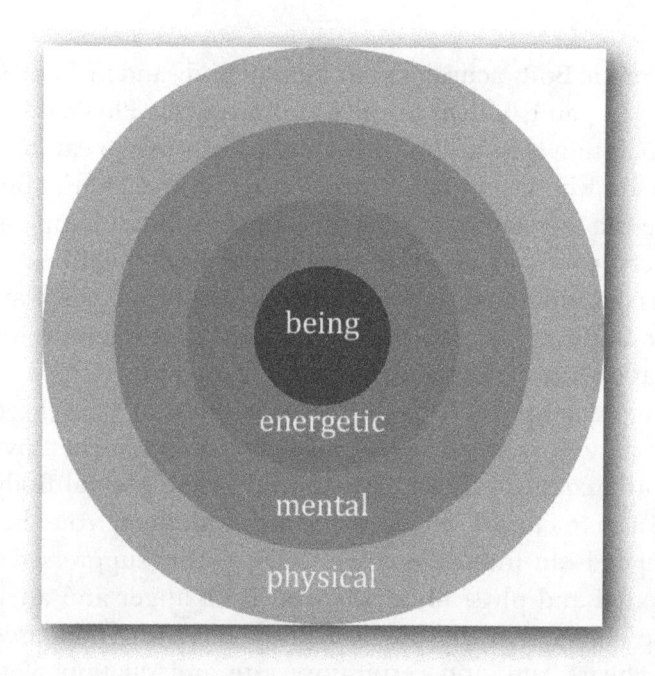

As we discover how to access the real experience of *being*, as opposed to understanding it on a diagram, we open the door to well-being. If we then follow through with actions that cultivate and balance The Three Bodies, well-being is realized. Your Energetic, Mental, and Physical Bodies then express fully, creatively, and powerfully as you choose. The Three Bodies are recognized as your forms—ways of describing you—yet you remain undivided and whole, as you always have been, a masterpiece beyond all boundaries and concepts.

Key Points

- You are *being* itself, expressing through Three Bodies—Physical, Mental, and Energetic.
- We are all interconnected within ourselves and with our environment through our Three Bodies.

MICHELANGELO'S MEDICINE

- <u>The Three Bodies</u> can be recognized, experienced, and explored through established introspective methods (see the activity following the Q&A).
- Medical science has primarily mapped only the Physical Body, and therefore it inevitably squeezes all of you into a physical anatomical model.
- The limited ability of medical science to cure many diseases is partially due to an incomplete understanding of human anatomy.

Q&A

- *Q: Is the anatomy of <u>The Three Bodies</u> as distinct as physical anatomy?*
  A: Physical anatomy is distinct because our minds have been trained to recognize it since childhood. The subtler anatomy of the Mental and Energetic Bodies is just as distinct when we learn to recognize it.
- *Q: Does your description of human anatomy contradict what science already knows?*
  A: No. <u>The Three Bodies</u> complement and complete what science already knows about the personal Physical Body.
- *Q: What is the line that divides one body from the next?*
  A: Your own awareness of <u>The Three Bodies</u> determines the dividing line. The Physical Body flows from the Mental Body, which flows from the Energetic Body. All three are unique processes within *being*. The contents of each body described in this chapter are landmarks from which to begin your own exploration. Ultimately, there is no dividing line, although it is useful to draw boundaries for the purposes of understanding and developing applications.
- *Q: Can I recognize <u>The Three Bodies</u> right now?*
  A: The main obstacle to recognizing your Three Bodies is the preconceived notion that you are primarily a physical structure. This notion acts like a veil in the Mental Body, obscuring the recognition of deeper aspects of the mind, the Energetic Body, and *being*. Seeing beyond that veil can be immediate or it may take time. It depends on how firmly preconceived notions are

entrenched and how willing a person is to practice established introspective methods. (You can begin with the activity following this Q&A.) Once you see through the dogma and step into adventure, your own experience can carry you swiftly.

- *Q: How can an understanding of The Three Bodies help me experience well-being?*

A: It is not the understanding of The Three Bodies alone that leads to well-being but the exploration and experience of them. Exploring The Three Bodies gives you the bona fide experience of what you have known in the corners of your mind for all your life—that you are much more than a collection of organs wrapped in skin. It also reveals that well-being can't be compartmentalized into *one* body, *my* body, or *your* body. Our bodies are entwined with the environment and all of nature. With this recognition comes a change in the behaviors we choose.

- *Q: How can The Three Bodies be incorporated into a true health care system?*

A: The first step is for researchers, clinical staff, and patients to begin exploring their Three Bodies. Book knowledge cannot substitute for direct knowledge of what we are made of and what well-being truly is. The next step will be to map our subjective experiences scientifically and develop a Science of Well-Being, which we will explore later in this book. The Science of Well-Being should be taught throughout the educational system at different levels, from grade school through graduate and medical school, so that tomorrow's society is more knowledgeable, more capable, and more well. A scientific understanding of The Three Bodies can be used to recognize and develop new, less invasive, more comprehensive technologies for diagnosis and treatment that engage the Mental and Energetic Bodies.

ACTIVITY:
Recognizing and Balancing The Three Bodies

Conscious breathing is a simple way to begin balancing <u>The Three Bodies</u>. Breathing can be easily accessed through the Physical Body while immediately connecting all Three Bodies.

1. Keep your eyes open. Take a few full, easy breaths and feel the movement of the abdomen and the flow of air through the nostrils. Feel your personal Physical Body moving.
2. Take a few full, easy breaths. Keep your eyes open and notice the environment around you. Notice the walls, the ceiling, and the floor. Notice the lights and the furniture. This is your extended Physical Body. It is made from the same material and came from the same place as your personal Physical Body.
3. Close your eyes. Take a few full, easy breaths. Notice your thoughts and feelings. Notice the memories and images that show up in your mind. Notice the internal commentary. Notice the difficulty or ease of this practice. Notice your desire to keep going or to quit. These constitute your Mental Body.
4. Take a few deeper breaths without straining yourself. Stay with the Mental Body. Allow any sense of discomfort to remain if it wishes, and to eventually move on. Allow the thoughts and feelings that rise up to pass by, as they please. Note that there is a silence between the uprisings. Rest in that silence. Old memories may flash by. Emotions may gush forth. Brilliant ideas may reveal themselves. Allow them, breathe with them, and again rest in silence. Eventually, you will feel an activation of energy—a charge. It may be faint. You may overlook it, doubt it, and question it. With sustained attention, it becomes unmistakable. This is just the edge of your Energetic Body. Keep breathing and balancing. The energy will become more noticeable. Explore steadily and responsibly. Rushing leads to imbalance and frustration. Going with the ebb and flow is the best route. Welcome to your Energetic Body.

5. Having recognized your Three Bodies, recognize that the divisions between them are not set in stone. Breathe and allow the divisions in your awareness to dissipate. Release constrictions. <u>The Three Bodies</u> are a representation of you, but are not all of you. You are undivided and whole. You are *being*.

If you would like to explore your Three Bodies further, an experiential course is offered at anoopkumar.com/journey

CHAPTER 8
What are the Four Pillars?

Completing my residency and moving back home to the Washington, DC, metropolitan area was a momentous occasion. A crucial part of my medical training had just ended, yet my career was just beginning. I was making decisions and calling the shots on my own without a more experienced set of eyes looking over my shoulder. Four years of residency training had prepared me well.

Completing residency also meant a decrease in work hours. That gave me the opportunity to explore what was possible for our medical treatment system. I had already developed some ideas of my own, but I wanted to know what the experts were saying.

I began reading everything I could get my hands on. First, I focused on the medical treatment system itself. I read about the intersection of policy and practice, the history of health care reform, and how our medical treatment system developed. I studied the business of medicine, the making of the medical consumer, and the push for quality and value in medicine. I researched the digital revolution, wellness, and integrative medicine.

There were so many topics to read about that I wondered how leaders in the industry kept abreast of everything. That question intrigued me, so I began analyzing the intersection of leadership and the medical treatment system. What were executives thinking about? How were they succeeding? How were they failing?

What I saw was organizational leaders putting out fires at the strategic level while clinicians did the same at the clinical level. I saw health care organizations struggling to tread water. I saw rampant use of terms like *innovation* and *out-of-the-box thinking* applied to very *still-in-the-box* strategies and programs. I saw that, even as they endeavored to help patients, executives, managers, and clinicians were often unwell themselves. Most profoundly, I saw that many of us in the system were trying to avoid these truths.

This gave me pause. I had to look in the mirror. As much as I was thinking about and cultivating well-being in my own way, my life was haphazard. In residency, I had developed poor lifestyle habits. I had to make a change. I started by renewing my focus on nutrition.

The steady diet of pizza and chicken wings I had developed over the prior few years gave way to more fresh fruits and vegetables. Within two days of making this change, I noticed an improvement in my energy level, mental clarity, and concentration. I got curious and decided to experiment further. I became vegan and even cut out the oil in my diet for a few months. I watched for my mind's response—it became clearer still, although my personal Physical Body grew weaker. Ultimately, I settled into a middle ground where I didn't fall into any particular category. Now, I'm not vegan, vegetarian, pescatarian, or paleo. I don't follow a specific diet. What works for me is eating plenty of fresh fruits and vegetables along with a moderate helping of what entices me.

Many times on this journey I've come to a crossroads where what I was learning and understanding was at odds with the practices in my own life. Each time I had to correct course so that I could keep going. I didn't want to experience well-being just once in a while. I wanted to develop it in my life and share it with others. I discovered that I could attain these goals by making choices in four key areas of life. These are <u>The Four Pillars</u> of well-being.

(1) CONNECTION – Connecting means getting in touch with all aspects of yourself. In the personal Physical Body, this takes the form of recognizing biological cues, such as hunger and pain, and responding appropriately. In the extended Physical Body, connecting means being in a setting you enjoy, with people whose company you enjoy. Connecting with others creates a community through the extended Physical Body that reinforces well-being.

In the Mental Body, connecting means becoming aware of your state of mind. It may include reflecting on your day, contemplating something that moved you, meditating, or any activity that turns your attention inward. Connecting with the Mental Body shifts your attention from the physical world to the mental one, ultimately allowing you to see that the boundary between the two is not set in stone.

In the Energetic Body, connecting means placing recognizing the battery—the charge—that underlies mental activity. It means seeing beyond (but not ignoring) the needs of the Physical Body and seeing beyond the hankerings of the Mental Body to the core of experience.

Ultimately, connecting is about simply *being*, which is the stillness beyond the activity of The Three Bodies. This is why connecting is the first pillar. It goes straight to the heart of well-being, anchoring the experience of well-being as it develops. It gives context to the remaining pillars. Amazingly, we have the ability to connect anywhere and anytime, even when he have only a few seconds available.

(2) NUTRITION – I'm tired of hearing the word *diet*. It has become so loaded that even hearing it is a turn-off to many people. Regardless of what the word may actually mean, the story around the word *diet* is that diets are hard, diets fail, and diets are fads. We could use the word *food* instead, but it's not specific enough.

What the body ultimately needs is not just any food—not just anything that will fit down your esophagus and make it to your stomach—but rather particular types of food. Specifically, the body is looking for nutrition. Nutrition gets to the heart of the issue. When your heart is beating over one hundred thousand times a day, never skipping a beat, what it requires is nutrition to keep it humming.

So what are the basics of nutrition? Many books and experts on nutrition offer conflicting advice. Some say avoid carbohydrates and stick with protein. Others say carbohydrates are good for you, but dairy should be avoided. Yet others say a balance of different kinds of foods is best. I can't make an official recommendation on what you should eat, because you are unique, but I can tell you this. What is good for you can't be based solely on expert recommendations, because you are not an "average" person. In fact, nobody is an average person.

Recommendations are based on studying populations over time and discovering what *generally* works. Yet, you are not a generalization. So the variety of expert recommendations actually makes sense because a person with a particular personality, body type, and metabolism will have an inclination toward particular foods. They may also be allergic to certain foods. What works best for you will be unique. It will make you feel good—not just when it's in your mouth and your tongue is singing but after it is digested and for hours to days afterward.

Having said that, I do think there is a simple nutritional rule of thumb that most people could follow to move them in the right direction: Eat more fresh fruits and vegetables with every meal and fewer processed foods, including sugar and salt. This alone will likely produce a noticeable change in how you feel.

We've talked about nutrition in terms of what you eat so far, but nutrition is much more than that. In the Mental Body, the thoughts you entertain are nutrition. The books you read and the shows you watch are nutrition. The conversations you partake of are nutrition. Just as consuming high-quality food will increase your well-being, engaging the Mental Body with high-quality content will also increase well-being.

In the Energetic Body, nutrition is the boost that comes from sustaining attention on the charge beyond the Physical and Mental Bodies. The energetic boost doesn't necessarily translate to a flurry of external activity, but rather to a revving up of the body's balancing process. This revving up naturally leads to the next pillar: movement.

(3) MOVEMENT – Movement replaces *exercise*, another loaded word. Yes, exercise is important, but at some point the word itself became an obstacle—something daunting that we *have* to do for sixty minutes at least four times a week (at least until the next study comes along and changes it up yet again).

Setting goals is important, but it's more important to simply start and do something. If you're not up to doing it three or four times a week, start with *something* today. Then build on that. Exercise can be strenuous, but it can also be simple and low key. *Movement* captures both beautifully. Stretch, stand up, touch your toes, take a few deep breaths—all movement counts.

Movement also applies to the Mental Body. Creatively expressing your ideas is *moving* your ideas, as opposed to letting them stagnate and atrophy. Being able to feel the emotions that pass through you and find avenues for their expression is also movement. This is one of the areas where our society has stagnated the most. In our schools, we teach our children the importance of intellectual movement by teaching a variety of subjects. We teach the importance of physical movement through physical education and play time. But we don't teach the importance or practice of emotional movement nearly as well. This has created a society that is emotionally undeveloped and out of balance. This imbalance inevitably moves from the Mental Body into the Physical Body, potentially manifesting as an array of mental and physical symptoms for which we cannot identify a cause.

In the Energetic Body, movement refers to allowing the flow of energy to circulate from the Energetic Body to the Mental and Physical Bodies. Remember that <u>The Three Bodies</u> are ways of organizing and understanding the human being. In practice, each body is continuously interfacing with the other two. As the Energetic Body begins to move and circulate, it clears stagnant beliefs and unexpressed emotions from the Mental Body. This clearing may be experienced as the recollection of old memories, the upwelling of emotions that haven't been felt for years, and also as joyfulness and clarity. As the circulation of energy continues, it will also change the Physical Body. Areas of tightness can relax, and pain can be alleviated or disappear completely. As muscles relax, your posture may spontaneously change.

Allowing the Energetic Body to move is like cleaning house. It cleans out and aligns the Mental and Physical Bodies, keeping <u>The Three Bodies</u> in balance.

(4) REST – This includes sleep and good ol' R&R, such as curling up with a good book. Both activate the restful state, turning off the stress response and promoting restoration. In today's to-do-list society, *rest* can be a bad word, especially at work. But "downtime" is essential. Some people find that they are more productive when they schedule rest time into their workday.

When you give your body a break, it goes to work on itself, eliminating toxins, fighting infections, repairing injured tissue, and releasing hormones that promote development. During the day, we often unknowingly leave the restful state and enter the stressful state. In fact, just waking up in the morning and remembering an irritating experience from the previous day can trigger it.

An irritating memory can activate your stress response as a protective mechanism. Although your life is not in danger, your brain prepares itself for the worst, signaling your adrenal glands to secrete adrenaline. Your pupils dilate, your blood vessels constrict, your blood pressure increases, and your heart starts pumping faster, a system-wide reaction. Eventually, once the brain recognizes no real threat exists, <u>The Three Bodies</u> return to their normal restful state.

Over time, frequent episodes of the stress response can change our baseline state from a restful one to a stressful one. Meditation, modifying your breathing pattern, and taking mental time-outs are great ways to start resetting your physiology, allowing your body's processes and functions to enjoy the restful state. In this way, rest can also be a form of connection. With practice, you will spend a greater amount of each day in a restful, connected state, even as you are going about your day.

Initially, resting the Physical Body can bring the buzz of mental activity to the forefront. This is exactly what happens in the early stages of meditation, during which it is common for the following kinds of thoughts to surface in the Mental Body:

Am I doing this right?
This is hard.
I'm not feeling peaceful!

If you have thoughts that are anything like these, know that having such doubts is a symptom of progress, because it is natural for the mind to resist diving deeper. Its tendency is to keep the shield up. Eventually, such thoughts will dissipate and the Mental Body will come to rest.

When the Mental Body rests, the Energetic Body can come to the forefront. The first pillar, connection, helps us recognize the presence of this Energetic Body. The second pillar, nutrition, sustains that awareness. The third pillar, movement, removes blocks. All of these culminate in the fourth pillar—rest. Resting in the Energetic Body means staying connected with it, and continuing to allow it to move as it needs to.

By addressing The Four Pillars, we address the *well* in *well*-being. What it means to be *well* changes depending on the culture, time period, and person. Nutrition as we define it today isn't the same as nutrition two hundred years ago. My idea of nutritious food isn't the same as yours. In other words, wellness is relative. We can use The Four Pillars to approach what wellness means to us. But to experience well-being, we must also add *being* to wellness. *Being* is not relative. It is not fundamentally different in you and me. It only expresses differently through the The Three Bodies.

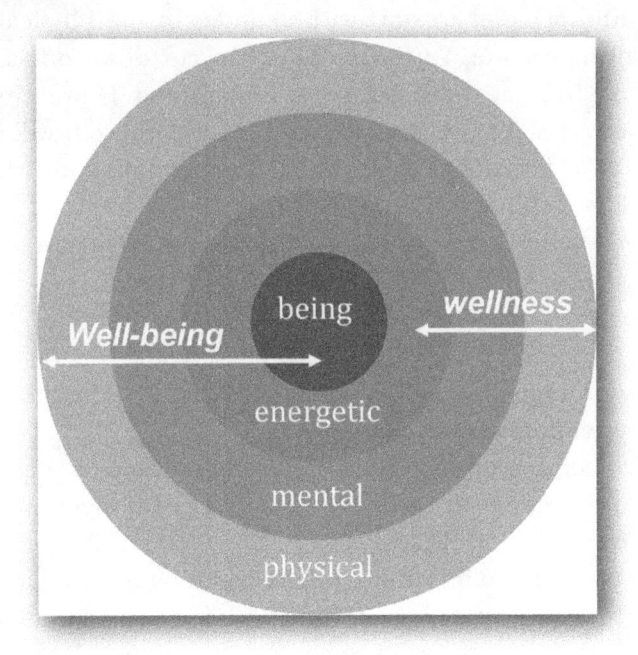

When we attend to The Four Pillars plus *being*, all other aspects of well-being will come into our line of sight. When you connect with yourself, you will become clear on what you want to spend your time on, which will begin to address occupational and social well-being. You will also be able to connect with others more easily. When you "move with yourself" and express yourself sincerely and effectively, your occupational, social, and even financial well-being may also be affected. And when you nourish yourself and rest, all of the above will be supercharged.

The knowledge we wish to see applied in the <u>medical treatment system</u> must first be recognized within ourselves. One step is all it takes to set the ball in motion. A concrete way to begin fortifying well-being in all areas of your life is to choose one of these four pillars and take one step today. If you are already acting on one or more pillars, continue that practice. If you desire, you can challenge yourself by choosing another pillar to explore. As more of us do this, we will reach a critical mass that the <u>medical treatment system</u> will have to accommodate.

Many find it easier to start with changes in the Physical Body, but each person is unique. You may choose to cut down on salt, go for a walk, squeeze in a nap, or meditate for ten minutes. However you choose to start, know that it's the perfect step for you, and so it will make a difference in your life and in the environment around you (which is your extended Physical Body, after all).

Your well-being is in your hands. You are the physician.

Key Points

- Any change you wish to see in the world starts within you. One step is all it takes to change.
- Well-being is an experience that is cultivated by making choices in four key areas—The Four Pillars: Connection, Nutrition, Movement, and Rest.
- *Connection* implies tuning in and listening to your Three Bodies.
- *Nutrition* is giving yourself nutritious food and a nourishing intellectual, emotional, and physical environment. It also means sustaining attention on the Energetic Body.
- *Movement* is moving the Physical Body, expressing your creative ideas, feeling and processing your emotions, and allowing your energy to flow throughout your bodies.
- *Rest* is getting enough downtime, getting sufficient sleep, and remaining balanced in the Energetic Body.

Part II
Transforming Health Care

CHAPTER 9
State of the Medical System

ealth care means different things to different people. To a patient, health care may signify pills and procedures, physicians, nurses, the clinic, the hospital, bills, and insurance companies. To a physician, it may suggest patients, the clinic, the hospital, academic journals, licensing exams, patient satisfaction scores, professional societies, and a paycheck. To a professional pundit, it may entail governmental regulations, lobbyists on Capitol Hill, and the latest round of policy. When two people are having a conversation about health care, it is not uncommon for each to have a different picture of what health care means, or a different focus and agenda.

Below is a diagram of health care's fundamental function—a patient receiving care from a practitioner.

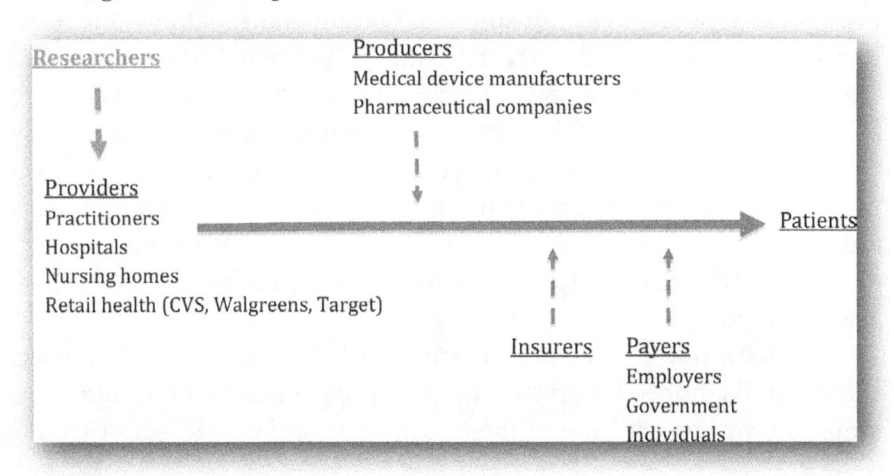

```
Researchers                Producers
    |                      Medical device manufacturers
    |                      Pharmaceutical companies
    ↓                          |
                               |
Providers                      ↓
Practitioners  ─────────────────────────────────→  Patients
Hospitals                          ↑         ↑
Nursing homes                      |         |
Retail health (CVS, Walgreens, Target)       |
                                Insurers   Payers
                                           Employers
                                           Government
                                           Individuals
```

The large arrow from left to right represents treatment delivery to the patient. This care is modified by four categories, shown as dotted vertical lines. Three of these four categories are well known. **Producers** manufacture the pharmaceuticals and medical devices that are the staples of hospitals and clinics. **Insurers** ideally make care affordable. **Payers** ensure that the system is funded, keeping the care delivery pipeline functioning. Then there's a fourth category: **Researchers**.

Researchers are the most powerful "suppliers" in the entire system, although they are not traditionally thought of as such. More than the supply of medicines or devices, it is the *supply of information* that has the greatest power to influence the system. In this sense, researchers are indeed suppliers in the value chain of care. They produce the research that creates medical science and molds the minds of clinicians and patients.

Generally, when we think of medical research, we picture research into new diseases and new drugs and procedures to fight those diseases. Why this singular focus on fighting disease? There are two reasons.

The first is habit. We are not used to thinking about health and well-being in health care. We're used to fighting disease. It's the model that's been handed down over decades. And we tend to do as we've always done. The second reason is money. Even if researchers think differently and start investigating the human body from new angles, they have to find funding to support that research. That can be difficult when producers invested in the disease-based model of medical treatment are the ones funding a large proportion of research studies. One study in the *New England Journal of Medicine* states that 70 percent of the clinical trials conducted in the United States are commissioned by private companies.[1]

Disease is the central hub of today's medical treatment system. I've heard people suggest that the system revolves around physicians, hospitals, and pharmaceutical companies, but these are actually symptoms of a disease-based focus. The way that disease is formally represented and defined in the medical treatment system is through the International Classification of Diseases, or ICD.

The ICD, now in its tenth iteration (ICD-10), has a list of over sixty thousand diagnoses. When you visit your physician with some ailment or symptom, you receive one of those sixty-thousand-plus diagnoses, along with its associated code. Based on that ICD-10 code, you or your insurance company receive a bill and your physician is reimbursed. That code becomes part of your medical history and connects all the moving parts of the <u>medical treatment system</u> revolving around you.

Every patient must have an ICD-10 code, even if it's something as generic as "Encounter for screening, unspecified." If you come to the ED with symptoms of abdominal distress and I evaluate your pain, ultimately concluding that it's not appendicitis, cholecystitis, a bowel obstruction, a heart attack (sometimes masked by abdominal pain), or a host of other emergency conditions, we may decide together that the plan of care is for you to rest at home and follow up with your physician. At the end of that visit to the ED, I'm obliged to assign you an ICD-10 code, just as any clinician in any <u>healing system</u> might assign you a diagnosis. To satisfy this requirement, I look for the diagnosis that best represents the reason you came to the ED. That diagnosis may well be "abdominal pain, generalized."

I remember the first time this happened in medical school. I asked my supervising physician what the diagnosis would be for a patient I had evaluated with abdominal pain. Though the cause eluded me, I had eliminated the possible emergencies. "What does the patient have?" he asked me.

"I'm not sure. I don't know what he has."

"Why is he here?"

"Abdominal pain."

"There you go. The diagnosis is abdominal pain."

I found this extremely odd. The patient was going home with a *symptom* that now was his *diagnosis*. He could've made the same diagnosis at home (although he would certainly risk missing something much more serious). How can we turn symptoms into diagnoses simply to satisfy a bookkeeping system?

There are two answers. First, in the ED, the clinical team and diagnostic equipment are oriented toward diagnosing and managing life-threatening emergencies first and foremost, as they should be. Once we know the patient is safe and his or her symptoms have been managed as well as possible in the ED, the focus shifts to the next phase to further investigate the patient's condition—whether that's in the hospital, at home, or with his or her primary care physician.

The second answer is that medical science has a remarkably incomplete understanding of disease, its causes, and its manifestations. Specifically, clinicians in most hospitals are constrained to working mainly at the level of the Physical Body. While it is appropriate for clinicians to stay within their scope of practice, the medical treatment system is failing patients when it doesn't harness the useful, practical knowledge in every healing system around the world. The availability of that knowledge depends on medical research, again demonstrating why researchers are the most powerful suppliers in the health care value chain.

Because medical research primarily focuses on the Physical Body, with less research on the Mental Body and even less on the Energetic Body, the medical treatment system today is centered on the allopathic healing system. *Allopathy* is not a common word in most medical circles, yet it is one of the most powerful concepts in the medical treatment system.

The word *allopathy* was coined by Samuel Hahnemann to distinguish between two different approaches to medical treatment. The healing system that Hahnemann created, homeopathy, was based on the principle that "like cures like." (The root *homeo* means *similar*, or *like*.) This is not unlike the principle we use today to develop vaccinations: Small, attenuated doses of a substance that would otherwise cause illness are given to boost the immune system, which then resists the full-blown illness.

The root *allo* means *other*. *Allopathy* therefore refers to a healing system in which the medicine given is *other than* or in opposition to the symptoms of illness. The general idea is that homeopathy aims to boost the immune system while allopathy aims to directly counteract the symptoms or causative agent.

Allopathy is the particular healing system in which I, along with most other physicians you will encounter in most hospitals, am trained. Allopaths are generally trained to see diseases as processes of the Physical Body, even in the case of mental illness. It makes sense that when a disease manifests as an emergency on the physical level, allopathy is a good bet, especially if the patient has suffered acute trauma, a severe infection, or any other condition that is an impending threat to life. Allopathy's greatest strengths lie in treating these kinds of disease.

The shortcomings of allopathy are also well known, especially when it comes to chronic disease. On every shift I see patients in the ED returning with worsening symptoms of hypertension, diabetes, heart disease, cancer, respiratory disease, and autoimmune disease. The approach to treatment in all of these cases is to *manage* the symptoms. There is little talk about *curing* the underlying causes. This is partly because of a lack of understanding of the Mental and Energetic Bodies and how they influence the Physical Body. In some cases, these chronic problems can be alleviated by a deeper understanding and experience of The Three Bodies, as well as renewed focus on The Four Pillars.

Healing systems other than allopathy have collectively been referenced as *alternative* or *complementary medicine*, with allopathy being called *conventional medicine*. These are generic terms that were useful decades ago but are no longer informative.

For example, traditional Chinese medicine is not strictly either alternative or conventional. For some people it is conventional, and for others it is an alternative, depending on the person and the clinical context. Allopathy, too, is not strictly conventional or alternative; it is simply allopathy. In the context of certain types of back pain, allopathy may be an alternative and shiatsu or Thai massage may be conventional, whereas in cases of acute trauma, allopathy is likely to be conventional.

The question of "convention" should be determined by the specific clinical context, not tradition. In other words, the unique circumstances of each medical case should be the determining factor in whether the "conventional" approach is primary or secondary. It's time to leave the antiquated jargon behind.

All healing systems, including allopathy, need more and better medical research. We must research each healing system in depth, with careful consideration and understanding of its tenets, particularly focusing on the strengths and weakness of each one. Equipped with this knowledge, we need to further research the best way to bring them all together to form a true and complete health care system.

We are making some progress on this front, but have yet to find a common framework that accommodates the unique mechanisms of each healing system. This is because the anatomical schema used by some healing systems employ a different perspective of the human body. Systems such as Ayurveda and traditional Chinese medicine have recognized and appreciated the Mental and Energetic Bodies for millennia, but Western medical science hasn't yet found a way to rationally reconcile those bodies with the Physical Body. (We will explore a way to do this in a subsequent chapter.)

When we don't understand how a system works, it can make it difficult to test its effectiveness, because the method of observation, or the method of testing, may interfere with or affect the very mechanism that allows the system to work. This is why we try to account for the placebo effect in clinical trials, yet we do so incompletely because we do not yet know the mechanism by which the placebo effect works.

The placebo effect is often dismissed as an improvement in the patient's experience simply due to "belief." There is often no further inquiry into how exactly belief translates into changes in the Physical Body. That question will remain difficult to answer as long as we are stuck in a physical model of the human being. As we learn more about The Three Bodies, the mechanism of the placebo effect will become clearer. Instead of trying to eliminate placebo effects from treatment, we will then find ways to begin to harness them. Only then will we develop the knowledge required to fully evaluate all healing systems around the world and find a way to integrate them in a true, complete health care system.

Key Points

- Researchers are the most powerful suppliers in the health care value chain because they supply the science that molds the minds of patients and clinicians.
- Allopathic medical treatment focuses on disease because its science is focused on disease. The nature of life and well-being remain a scientific blind spot.
- Every healing system has its own name—allopathy, Ayurveda, homeopathy, chiropractic, and so on. The generic terms *alternative, complementary,* and *conventional medicine* are nonspecific and antiquated.
- Understanding the Mental and Energetic Bodies will yield new insight into the mechanism of placebo and how to harness it for healing.

Q&A

- *Q: Don't all healing systems focus on disease?*
  A: All healing systems recognize disease. But many healing systems also recognize and study subtler life processes in the Mental and Energetic Bodies. In those systems, restoring order in the life processes is the focus, not attacking the disease. This offers a different kind of benefit.
- *Q: What do you think of the phrase "integrative medicine"?*
  A: It's an accurate description of what medicine should be—the best of all healing systems applied to a specific clinical context. Once medicine truly becomes an integrative practice, we will be able to drop the adjective *integrative*. It will simply be medicine—what works.
- *Q: How can you value all healing systems equally when allopathy has the most evidence supporting it?*
  A: We study what we know to study. If we don't explore and experience the Mental and Energetic Bodies, we won't understand how to study them. For example, what we try to weed out of studies as placebo effects are partly the result of mechanisms in the Mental and Energetic Bodies. The evidence we currently have, and our understanding of it, is therefore remarkably incomplete.

References

1. T. Bodenheimer, "Uneasy Alliance: Clinical Investigators and the Pharmaceutical Industry," *New England Journal of Medicine* 342:1539–44.

CHAPTER 10
What is the Informational Problem?

When I made a recent trip to San Diego for a conference, I didn't have to worry about taking a map. The global positioning system (GPS) on my smartphone got me to my hotel. But what would have happened if the GPS had relied on outdated information? I remember using my GPS app to navigate to a restaurant once. After a few turns, it proclaimed, "You have reached your destination." But I wasn't at my destination. I was facing a dead end.

The same is happening in medical care today. Our map of the human body is outdated. To better understand this, let's organize medical care into two branches.

1. The informational branch—what we *know* about the human body
2. The operational branch—what we *do* to help patients

What we know about the human body is informational in nature. Medical research has created a large repository of information. The power of that information is that we can act on it to help patients. In other words, that information must be operationalized, put to use.

The informational branch features two main categories—medical research and medical science. Medical research is an ongoing activity of international scope; hundreds of billions of dollars are poured into it every year. Scientists around the world conduct studies in the hopes of discovering the next great cure or wonder drug. Although medical research is an essential activity of medical science, I choose to define medical science distinctly. For our purposes, medical science is the cumulative knowledge that has been accepted, based on medical research.

The operational branch includes the factors that influence how we apply the information coming from medical research and science. Almost every issue that experts talk about when it comes to improving medical treatment is operational. This includes insurance coverage, access to care, cost of care, incentivizing performance, and tort reform.

A good way to think about the two branches of medical care, informational and operational, is to visualize a wheel. The hub of the wheel is informational—everything we know about health and disease. The spokes of the wheel are operational, carrying the information that we know to medical care professionals, then to patients on the perimeter of the wheel, where clinical care is implemented. The informational and operational branches are complementary and keep medical care running, just as a hub and its spokes stabilize the wheel.

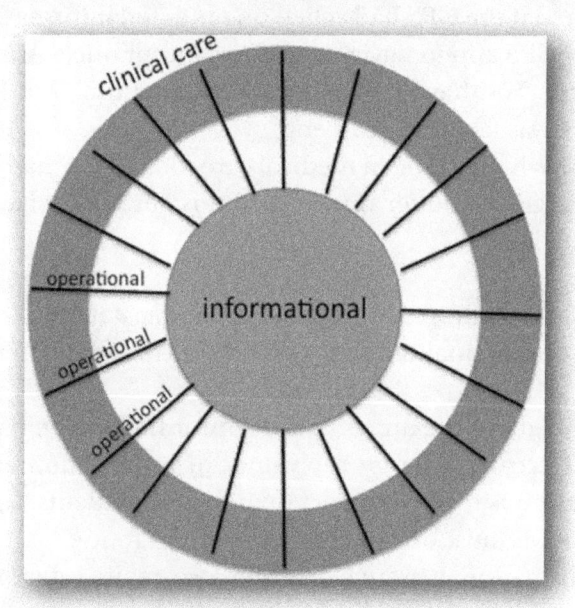

For example, medical research has shown that asthma—an inflammatory condition of the airways—responds to treatment with bronchodilators (which open up the airways) and steroids. This is the informational component at the hub of wheel. That information becomes operationalized when its application in the clinical setting is subjected to an onslaught of other factors, including insurance coverage and access to care, the spokes of the wheel. After making its way through that operational maze, it reaches the patient at the periphery of the wheel.

Given this categorization, we can identify two types of problems in today's medical care—again, informational and operational. Operational problems are well known. They're the ones that are commonly discussed on the news.

In 2009 and 2010, there was a great deal of talk about the operational problems in the context of medical care reform and the Affordable Care Act. I was in residency at the time and remember catching snippets of the heated words exchanged over universal health insurance. Ultimately, the idea of a single-payer system fell through, but it wasn't the first time it had been considered, by a long shot. Operational problems such as these have been discussed in various iterations of medical care reform since the early 1900s.

We have mounted a frontal attack on the operational problems in medical care, with varying degrees of success. It thrills me to see that people are dedicating themselves to solving these problems, but it also gives me pause. My work in the ED has shown me that in many cases we are unable to help patients in a meaningful way beyond suppressing their symptoms because we simply don't have the information that tells us how.

I remember a young patient who came to the ED with terrible abdominal cramping and diarrhea. For the past six years she had been dealing with inflammatory bowel disease. Initially, her flare-ups had occurred once or twice a year, but now they were every other month. She feared eating because she never knew which meal might trigger her symptoms.

From a clinical perspective, there appeared to be no acute life threat, but it was obvious that this patient was at her wit's end. She had been through medical treatment cycles many times before and, providing her evaluation in the ED didn't turn up anything unexpected, she knew what to expect in the end—pain pills, a potent anti-inflammatory medication, dietary recommendations, and follow-up visits with her gastroenterologist and primary care physician.

By the end of her stay in the ED, my patient was feeling a little better, but *a little better* just isn't good enough. In this case (and many others like it), the treatment we provide is important, but not effective enough. Why don't we know more?

The most pervasive problem we have in medical care today is not operational. No matter how much progress we make, we can't change the fact that operational problems are the spokes of the wheel. They will always convey the information of medical research and medical science from the hub. Solving only the operational problems in medical care would be like running a restaurant that is humming on all cylinders, yet consistently serving stale food.

Operational problems make the news and thus capture most of the public's attention. This has allowed the Informational Problem to become the most dominant and pervasive problem in medical care, while remaining essentially out of sight. To bring health and well-being to the medical treatment system, we must shine a light on the Informational Problem.

There are two parts to the Informational Problem—medical research and medical science. Problems with medical research are well documented. Here are the opinions of two prominent medical voices:

> ...much of the scientific literature, perhaps half, may simply be untrue. Afflicted by studies with small sample sizes, tiny effects, invalid exploratory analyses, and flagrant conflicts of interest, together with an obsession for pursuing fashionable trends of dubious importance, science has taken a turn towards darkness.[1]
> — RICHARD HORTON, EDITOR OF LANCET

> ...similar conflicts of interest and biases exist in virtually every field of medicine, particularly those that rely heavily on drugs or devices. It is simply no longer possible to believe much of the clinical research that is published, or to rely on the judgment of trusted physicians or authoritative medical guidelines. I take no pleasure in this conclusion, which I reached slowly and reluctantly over my two decades as an editor of The New England Journal of Medicine.[2]
> —MARCIA ANGELL, SENIOR LECTURER AT HARVARD MEDICAL SCHOOL

As a physician who has dedicated a large part of his life to patient care, I find quotes like these hard to take. Am I not that trusted physician that Marcia Angell referred to? Is my judgment impaired? Hearing that a significant part of what I've been taught about clinical treatment is based as much or more on profit than on impartial research is frankly painful, although not surprising. Most physicians, including myself, acknowledge this problem and talk about it, even while continuing to prescribe medications as we were taught to. These are difficult, uncomfortable issues that deserve our full attention. They pertain not just to rarely used drugs and medical devices but also to some of the most popular prescriptions on the market.

If up to half of the medical research is tainted, should we all simply stop taking our medications? No, because over time our bodies grow accustomed to pharmacological therapies; suddenly stopping certain drugs cold turkey can be life-threatening. A good example is common blood pressure medication. These drugs alter the body's physiology so that the blood vessels are no longer tightly constricted, thus reducing blood pressure. But suddenly cutting off medication can cause the blood vessels to rebound, snapping back to an even more constricted state and spiking blood pressure to a new, higher baseline. Many other popular medicines have these same dangers.

The way forward is to diligently pursue more fundamental principles of well-being. As we cultivate well-being and our bodies begin to heal, we will be able to reduce the use of some medications and discontinue the use of others altogether, in conjunction with a clinician's advice. As much as we talk about the importance of lifestyle changes to improve our well-being, their effectiveness is still underestimated by the medical treatment system. As Drs. Dean Ornish and Caldwell Esselstyn have shown, lifestyle modifications are capable of reversing diabetes and even severe heart disease. We must educate ourselves on approaches like these that emphasize the importance of The Four Pillars.

Now we come to the core of the Informational Problem—medical science. Remember how we distinguished medical science from medical research for our purposes: medical science is what we know for sure, based on the findings of previous and ongoing medical research. This brings to mind a Mark Twain quote: "It ain't what you don't know that gets you into trouble. It's what you know for sure that just ain't so."

The biggest problem with medical science today is that it is outdated by at least one hundred years. That's not a typo. For over a century, we have known that all matter, including the physical human body, is made up of two constituents—particles and space.

Each atom that comprises our body is made up of these infinitesimal particles. When those particles are compared with the volume of the atom, we find that the atom is predominantly space, with only a trace of particles. In fact, space accounts for over 99.99 percent of an atom's volume, and therefore accounts for over 99.99 percent of our apparently solid physical body. Yes, greater than 99.99 percent of your body is space, not "stuff."

How can this be? After all, we can touch our physical bodies, right? They seem so solid. The answer is simple. How we perceive things is a function of how sensitive our instruments of perception are. A needle tip appears very narrow to the naked eye. But when we augment the power of our eyes with a microscope, we can see that the tip can also appear dull, even flat, on a much finer scale. Similarly, what feels solid can also be perceived as spacious if we augment our perception of the Mental and Energetic Bodies.

> *The atom is as porous as the solar system. If we eliminated all the unfilled space in a man's body and collected his protons and electrons into one mass, the man would be reduced to a speck just visible with a magnifying glass.[3]*
> — SIR ARTHUR EDDINGTON, ASTROPHYSICIST

But that's not the end of the story. When we zoom in even further, we find that even these microscopic particles are not solid. They are abstractions—excitations of a field, not the hard, solid stuff that matter appears to be.

> *Isolated material particles are abstractions, their properties being definable and observable only through their interaction with other systems.[4]*
> —NIELS BOHR, WINNER OF THE 1922 NOBEL PRIZE IN PHYSICS

The bottom line? The "structure" of the human being is essentially a mental and energetic structure, not a physical one. Every cell and atom in your body is essentially a unique formation of <u>energy</u>. Even the 99.99 percent of you that is space is full of energy, a fact known to modern physics.

Recall that <u>The Three Bodies</u> are an expression of you. Each body is a unique interpretation, sustained by energy. The Physical Body is unique because it allows us to function and transact in the physical world. Yet, when we zoom in closely enough, we find nothing (no-thing) solid there, only energy. The Mental Body is unique because it allows us to interface with others in the mental world of thoughts and emotions. Yet, those thoughts and emotions, too, are not solid, not physical. They are modifications of a more fundamental level of mind, or energy. The basic ingredient of all Three Bodies is energy. (In a later chapter, we will address the discrepancy between the scientific and experiential aspects of energy, and find a way to reconcile them.)

> *It followed from the special theory of relativity that mass and energy are both but different manifestations of the same thing—a somewhat unfamiliar conception for the average mind. Furthermore, the equation $E = mc^2$... showed that very small amounts of mass may be converted into a very large amount of energy and vice versa. The mass and energy were in fact equivalent...*[5]
>
> *The mass of a body is a measure of its energy content.*[6]
> —ALBERT EINSTEIN, WINNER OF THE
> 1921 NOBEL PRIZE IN PHYSICS

We are long overdue for a new understanding of human anatomy. To see your own body as only a physical structure is to limit yourself to a frozen section under the lens of a microscope, a snapshot. You are not a still picture. You are fluid. You are moving. You are changing with the environment within and around you.

These are not the properties of a rigid physical structure, but rather of energy and information that are constantly in flux. What we call *form* perceived by our eyes is an ongoing *activity* of energy and information exchange, interpreted through the human nervous system. When we take our attention away from the activity, we automatically superimpose form. When we place attention back on the activity, the appearance of form recedes.

To take an example, the form of a wave rising in the ocean is nothing but the aggregate activity of water droplets. If we focus our attention on the activity of individual droplets, the form of the wave will be less apparent. And when we focus our attention on the overall form of the wave itself, the activity of individual water droplets will seem to recede. What we see is what we focus on.

Similarly, when we focus our attention on the form of the Physical Body, the activity of the Mental and Energetic Bodies will be less apparent, which is what is happening in the medical treatment system. If we focus our attention on the activity of the Energetic and Mental Bodies, the illusion of a separate Physical Body will recede.

You typically won't find a conversation about this in medical school, because the biomedical model is based on biochemistry—atoms, molecules, and macromolecules—not on reconciling what physics has understood intellectually with our own direct experience. Biochemistry is taught by conceptualizing molecules and atoms as solid balls connected to each other with sticks, entirely leaving out the properties of energy, fields, and vibrations that are the essential nature of atoms. Hence, generations of physicians and researchers have been taught ball-and-stick medicine: physical atoms, physical cells, physical organs, and ultimately a physical you.

The problem is, you are not only a physical being. Physicality is only one interpretation. Medical science is outdated today because it takes that lone interpretation as a singular truth. This is the core of the Informational Problem, and it influences every single aspect of the medical care system.

> *The frank realization that physical science is concerned with a world of shadows is one of the most significant of recent advances.*[3]
>
> *It is difficult for the matter-of-fact physicist to accept the view that the substratum of everything is of mental*

> *character. But no one can deny that mind is the first and most direct thing in our experience, and all else is remote inference — inference either intuitive or deliberate.*[3]
> — Sir Arthur Eddington, astrophysicist

Ever get the feeling that the <u>medical treatment system</u> doesn't see all of you? That it doesn't *get* you? That's not just an operational problem. That's not just people being stressed out. That's the <u>Informational Problem</u>.

Physicians know there is more to the patient than the disease and its physical manifestations, but our limited science doesn't understand that perspective. It handcuffs our ability to systematize real care. Physicians are unwittingly caught in a no-man's-land between personal experience and incomplete intellectual concepts.

In medical school, we are trained to view the human body as a physical structure that becomes afflicted with physical disease. Even mental illness is often reduced to fluctuations in neurotransmitters. We simply have not accessed the science needed to go beyond this basic understanding. That limitation shows up every time you get medical care.

What are the implications?

If the human body is thought of as a physical structure, then we look for physical explanations, physical diagnoses, and physical treatments. When rheumatoid arthritis flares up, we look for and find *things* called cytokines causing inflammation in the body, so we prescribe a pill that suppresses inflammation, not bothering to investigate a possible subtler explanation of and solution to inflammation.

To learn more about the body, we cut it up into small bits and see how they work together—the basis of reductionist and mechanistic thinking. If the human body is also seen as a mental and energetic structure, new possibilities emerge in the field of diagnosis and treatment at the level of mind and energy, including light, sound, meditation, and many other applications that are so far poorly understood.

Recognizing the energetic nature of the body is not *reducing* the body to energy. I am not suggesting that the body must be seen as only energy. Depending on the lens we choose to look through, the body can be interpreted as physical, mental, energetic, or an expression of *being* itself. Each lens provides a unique perspective on diagnosis and treatment. We must develop the versatility and vision to view health and disease from many angles. If we look for physicality only and turn a blind eye to energy, for example, it follows that we won't find evidence for energetic treatments. We see only what we have been trained to see.

Earlier, I gave an example of this medical myopia, noting first that ancient Chinese depictions of the human body missed the details of musculature, instead focusing on energetic pathways. The Western mind, on the other hand, depicts the same human body with an intricate musculature, altogether missing energetic pathways. This is how cultural bias and tradition hamper our full understanding of the human body.

Most medical researchers today have not been trained to perceive the mind or energy. It is no surprise that we continue to practice ball-and-stick medicine. If we dedicate resources to training our minds to consider a greater range of anatomy, including The Three Bodies, many of today's incurable diseases will be brought within the reach of medicine.

Key Points

- The medical treatment system has two aspects to it—operational and informational. We usually hear about operational issues (cost, coverage, access) and not the Informational Problem.
- The Informational Problem is the most pervasive and influential problem in the medical treatment system.
- The Informational Problem has two parts—poor-quality medical research and the false belief that the human body is primarily a physical structure.

References

1. Richard Horton, "What Is Medicine's 5-sigma?" http://www.thelancet.com/pdfs/journals/lancet/PIIS0140-6736%2815%2960696-1.pdf. Accessed 2/15/16.
2. Marcia Angell, "Drug Companies and Doctors: A Story of Corruption," http://www.nybooks.com/articles/2009/01/15/drug-companies-doctorsa-story-of-corruption/. Accessed 2/15/16.

3. Eddington, Arthur Stanley (1928). The Nature of the Physical World.
4. Bohr, Niels (1934). Atomic Theory and the Description of Nature. Ox Bow Press.
5. Atomic Physics (1948) by the J. Arthur Rank Organisation, Ltd.
6. Einstein, A. (1905). Does the Inertia of a Body Depend Upon Its Energy Content?

CHAPTER 11
What is Energy?

> *As a man who has devoted his whole life to the most clear headed science, to the study of matter, I can tell you as a result of my research about atoms this much: There is no matter as such.*[1]
> — MAX PLANCK, NOBEL PRIZE-WINNING PHYSICIST

One evening I walked into a room in the ED and greeted Mr. Wilkes, a smiling gentleman in his eighties. He was lying back on the stretcher and had a brown fedora on his head, the front tipped forward, covering his eyes. Below the brim of his hat, wrinkles extended downward like dry streams on a riverbed. He wore a faded azure shirt tucked into brown pants, which were held up by suspenders.

He had come to the ED to "get his legs checked out," and had done me the courtesy of rolling up his pant legs to the knees. On the floor next to the stretcher was a pair of worn-out loafers, stuffed with his socks. He seemed like someone who was making a brief pit stop, as though he had somewhere else to be very soon.

It was quickly apparent why Mr. Wilkes had come in. Both of his legs were swollen, the skin tight and reddish. Yet the smiling gentleman seemed generally unconcerned by this while I went about taking a history and doing a physical exam. He happily answered any questions I had and kept repeating, "I just want to know what's going on. That's all." Then he'd smile.

He was moving his legs freely and without pain. There was no suggestion of trauma. I checked the pulses in his feet. No problems there. Infection was a possibility, although it would be unusual for him to simultaneously develop an infection in both lower legs, especially when he hadn't been having any problems with them before.

I informed Mr. Wilkes that I'd be ordering a couple tests and would be back to check on him. When the ultrasound report came back, I wasn't surprised at the results. It confirmed that he had blood clots in both legs, extending from the calves into the upper thighs. To this day, I have not seen another patient with such extensive blood clots in both legs. I couldn't figure out why he had them. He didn't have any of the typical risk factors, although an underlying malignancy was a distinct possibility.

The real danger was that one of these blood clots could break free and make its way through the bloodstream to his lungs, likely getting stuck as the vessels narrowed. Given the extent of the clots, such a pulmonary embolism could prove fatal. If he'd had fewer and smaller blood clots, he could've been treated as an outpatient. But not in this case.

I explained this diagnosis to Mr. Wilkes, telling him that he should be admitted to the hospital and put on blood thinners. Immediately. He was still smiling.

"Thanks, doc, but I'm ready to go."

Go where? Home? Heaven? I was sure he misunderstood. "Mr. Wilkes, what I'm saying is that there is an extremely high risk of these blood clots going to your lungs, making it very difficult for you to breathe, and dropping your blood pressure to life-threatening levels. You could die."

"I know, doc. We all gotta go sometime."

I couldn't understand. He appeared to be in relatively good health, although perhaps he knew something I didn't. If we treated the blood clots it was reasonable to expect that he could live well for quite a bit longer. I inquired further about his reason for choosing no treatment. Why did he come in for a diagnosis if he was not going to do anything about it? It puzzled me.

After another five minutes of conversation, I was convinced that Mr. Wilkes wasn't going to change his mind. He wanted to go home, spend time with his dog, and let whatever happened happen, even if that were a life-threatening pulmonary embolism. Reluctantly, I discharged Mr. Wilkes from the ED against medical advice. He happily signed the papers, smiled at me, and left the ED on his swollen legs.

As a student of pathophysiology, I didn't agree with Mr. Wilkes's decision, but as his physician I didn't have a choice. His decision was based on what he valued most—being at home, even if it could cost him his life.

I sometimes think back and wonder how Mr. Wilkes saw himself. Maybe he knew there was more to him than his Physical Body. After all, he apparently wasn't that concerned about it. Perhaps he saw himself as something more—as mind or as spirit. Or perhaps he didn't think about any of that. Maybe he was simply a person who lived life as it came, and went. I never had the chance to ask him.

If I could talk to Mr. Wilkes now, I would. I wonder what he'd say if I suggested that our medical treatment system needed to start seeing its patients in a new light. I wonder what he'd say if I suggested that his body was not merely a physical structure but an energetic structure. I'm not sure, but I feel as though he'd smile again now as he did then.

The idea that we are energetic beings is not a new one. Perhaps the best example of the energetic model in American medicine is the work of Martha Rogers, RN, PhD. In her brilliant work "An Introduction to the Theoretical Basis of Nursing," Rogers described the entire human being as an "irreducible, indivisible ... energy field identified by pattern and manifesting characteristics that are specific to the whole and which cannot be predicted from knowledge of the parts."[2]

Rogers describes a continuity of the human being with the environment, using the model of an energy field. Her work is arguably the most overlooked book in medical care today. It is not just a theoretical basis of nursing, but of all medicine and all healing systems.

Variations of Rogers's model have been around for centuries. In AD 780, the Indian poet-philosopher Shankara described the continuity of the human being with the environment using a model of consciousness.

This model depicts the essential nature of the human being as consciousness, sometimes referred to as *being*, or *awareness*. Here, consciousness does not refer to subtypes, such as human consciousness or animal consciousness. Rather, it refers to the very principle of existence.

ANOOP KUMAR, MD

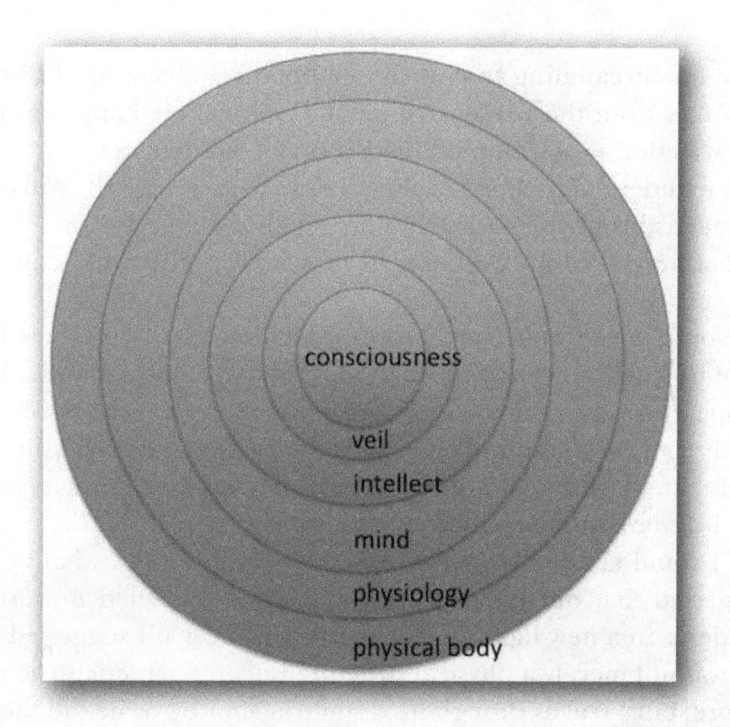

Diagram: concentric circles labeled from center outward: consciousness, veil, intellect, mind, physiology, physical body.

The physical body, physiology, mind, and other concentric circles in the diagram are progressive layers, appearing to be different from consciousness only because of a limitation in awareness, or a veil. If we superimpose The Three Bodies on this model, the personal Physical Body would be the outermost ring, the Mental Body would include mind and intellect, and the Energetic Body would be between the intellect and consciousness.

India's ancient medical system of Ayurveda (*ayur* = life, *veda* = knowledge) is also based on a theory of energy. It classifies the human being as a combination of three energies: the energy of movement is *vata* (wind), the energy of transformation is *pitta* (fire), and the energy of structure is *kapha* (earth).

If we look to China, the model of the human being is based on the five elements of fire, earth, wood, metal, and water, and the vital energy of *chi*, which flows through a system of meridians.

In the United States, chiropractic is based on a philosophy of vital energy that can be blocked based on the position of the vertebral column relative to the nerves that pass through it.

In cultures around the world, as well as here in the United States, there has been a long-standing appreciation for and understanding of the body as something other than physical. Some see a vital energy or life force that runs through the body. Others see the body itself as an energetic structure or function, or as an expression of a more fundamental consciousness. Medical science has systematically struck down ideas of vitalism and metaphysics over the decades because of its demand for a purely physical model of the human being. Yet we know that the physical model itself is an interpretation of something fundamentally nonphysical.

In today's society, we think about <u>energy</u> in many different ways. One of the most common is the global energy crisis, generally recognized as the depletion of Earth's natural resources (specifically fossil fuels, including oil, coal, and natural gas). We also think of energy in terms of light from the sun, which drives the process of photosynthesis. In the human body, we think about energy in the form of a molecule called adenosine triphosphate, or ATP. When a molecule of ATP breaks apart, energy is released that is used to power the reactions in the body. These examples are objective, measurable forms of energy, or *veritable energy*.

But energy can also be subjective. Thoughts are energy. The thought energy that an executive team puts into a strategic planning session results in the actions they take to implement their strategy. Emotions are energy. Just ask any coach motivating his team for the big game's second half. And the body is energy. Every particle in your body is a formation of energy.

Energy healers are able to subjectively detect energy. That type of energy is called *putative energy*—energy that we are not able to comprehensively measure. Some call it *chi*, some call it *prana*, some simply call it *energy*, and some don't name it at all. Because it's not yet measurable, critics contend that such subtle types of energy don't actually exist, meaning that they have no experience of it.

If we want to detect putative energy, we must first ensure that we are using the proper tools. If I want to see the furniture in an unlit room, I must know how to shine a flashlight on it. Similarly, if I want to detect putative energy, I must know how to train and direct my attention in such a way as to perceive it.

A more standard definition of energy that many of us learned in high school is that energy is *the ability to do work*. We can calculate energy using mathematical formulas, such as the ones for kinetic and potential energy. The units used to measure these forms of energy include joules (J), kilowatt-hours (kWh), and calories (cal).

The point is that there is no single definition or experience of energy, as much as we would like to nail it down with an objective measurement. Scientists have not yet figured out what energy fundamentally is, and as long as we consider only the objective aspect of energy, we never will.

> *It is important to realize that in physics today, we have no knowledge of what energy "is." We do not have a picture that energy comes in little blobs of a definite amount. It is not that way.*[3]
> — RICHARD FEYNMAN, THEORETICAL PHYSICIST, NOBEL PRIZE WINNER

What we call *energy* is a versatile activity that can be detected in different forms as a subjective experience and an objective measurement, depending on the lens we choose and the training we have. Our progress in medical science, and science in general, depends on our appreciating and studying both forms, as we will see in the next chapter.

Questioning physicality, or the physical-ness of the objects around us, is not new. It has been explored in areas such philosophy, metaphysics, and spirituality for millennia. It only sounds new because modern scientific culture is based on the presumption that the physical world is fundamental and mental and energetic experiences are secondary, if at all acknowledged. But when physics itself came to question physicality by discovering that physical objects can also be interpreted as forms of energy, the possibility for a new interpretation—or rather the possibility that millennia-old interpretations may be correct—once again arose.

> *Matter, too, has life; it is energy solidified.*[4]
> —ALBERT EINSTEIN, WINNER OF THE 1921 NOBEL PRIZE IN PHYSICS

You would think that the world would have taken notice, especially medical science, which has a responsibility to address disease, suffering, healing, and well-being. But that didn't happen. Why?

The most obvious reason is that the objects around us appear as physical structures. You and I may be made of energy, but we are not aware of that most of the time because our minds are attuned to the physical. Scientists may suspect that matter is a form of energy, but when they're eating a slice of their favorite pizza, they're not experiencing energy, they're experiencing pepperoni. The point is that how we interpret what is happening is based more on ingrained habits than on what science has demonstrated.

Imagine seeing a beautiful sunset at the beach. Our experience is that a glowing orb is slowly descending and setting beyond the ocean. Naturally, we call it a sunset. But intellectually we know that the sun does not set at all. The Earth is simply moving in such a way that the sun appears to be setting. Despite knowing that, we still call it a sunset and experience the sun setting. Habit often wins over fact. The scene you are a part of right now, including your own personal Physical Body, can be appreciated physically, mentally, or energetically. It is a matter of training the faculty of perception.

As much as we may intellectually understand that we are forms of energy, until we explore it, play with it, and experiment with it ourselves, the experience of energy will not take hold. It will remain a remote concept. No matter how much we may know the truth intellectually, our habitual experience overwhelms it, and the benefits of that understanding will not translate to the practical level of our daily lives.

The second reason that medical treatment continues to target the Physical Body is that a change in perception would challenge entrenched cultural norms and economic structures. Change at the systemic level takes persistence. If the body is a form of energy, then medical treatment consists of ... everything. Every-*thing* and every mental activity, being essentially energetic in nature, has the potential to influence the well-being of our own energetic system, positively or negatively. Light, sound, scent, touch, taste, all forms of radiation, the company we keep, the environment, our breathing, and pretty much anything else we name can be seen in a medical light.

Is an energetic model of the human body more than just a neat trick? Is there a therapeutic benefit to viewing the body as an energetic structure? Yes. Seeing the body as an energetic structure gives us much more information to work with. It opens up vaults of medical knowledge from cultures around the world. If we are able to translate the knowledge captured in all the <u>healing systems</u> around the world into the concepts and language of modern science, we will find opportunities to harness and develop those insights into cures for disease and new ways to support well-being.

The Institute of Noetic Sciences published a bibliography of over 3,500 documented spontaneous remissions of diseases, many of which were considered incurable cancers. Instead of ignoring or explaining these away as random or serendipitous, what if we could actually learn how to cure what has been considered incurable? The <u>medical treatment system</u> would be on its way to becoming a true <u>health care system</u>.

Harold Saxton Burr, PhD, a professor of anatomy at Yale University, conducted a series of experiments in the 1940s in which he detected and measured the electrical fields of humans, animals, and trees. He called these *life fields,* or *L-fields.* He found that the L-fields of trees varied predictably according to day/night cycles, lunar cycles, and the appearance of sunspots. By measuring changes in the electrical field in humans, he was able to predict the course of disease and healing.

In 1972, he wrote, "In the case of L-fields [life fields] there is no technical reason why their use by doctors should take so long. Modern instruments are reliable; and any intelligent man or woman can learn the techniques of taking and interpreting L-field readings in a short period of intensive instruction.... Immediate and practical results, in fact, can stem from this adventure in science...."[5]

Time and time again, we find evidence for an energetic basis of human anatomy, beginning thousands of years ago, solidified with the science of a hundred years ago, and verified in experiments in the decades since then. Yet, we have resisted embracing this model, leaving us bereft of a more complete <u>Science of Well-Being</u>. A more complete understanding of energy is the bridge we need to learn from the many pioneers whose vision has seemed too lofty for us to understand and implement.

Key Points

- The energetic basis of the human being has been recognized around the world for millennia.
- The relationship between energy and matter was discovered by modern science about one hundred years ago.
- Energy has two forms—veritable (objective) and putative (subjective).
- Bridging veritable and putative energy will yield a complete understanding of energy and is a step toward a Science of Well-Being.

Q&A

Q: Is the energy that scientists measure and the energy that healers feel the same energy?
A: They are aspects of the same subtle activity, expressing in different ways. Scientists measure the aspect of energy that is captured in the physical plane, while healers work with energy in the mental and energetic planes. More on this in the next chapter.

References

1. *Das Wesen der Materie* (*The Nature of Matter*), 1944 speech in Florence, Italy.
2. Rogers, M. E. (1991). An introduction to the theoretical basis of nursing. Philadelphia: Davis.
3. Feynman, R. P., Basic Books (Firm), & California Institute of Technology. (2003). The Feynman lectures on physics: Volume 1. New York: Basic Books.
4. Hermanns, W., & Einstein, A. (1983). Einstein and the poet: In search of the cosmic man. Brookline Village, MA: Branden Press.
5. Burr, H. S. (2000). Blueprint for immortality: The electric patterns of life. London: Saffron Walden.

CHAPTER 12
Why do we Need a Science of Well-Being?

It should come as no surprise that the solution to the Informational Problem in the medical treatment system is better information and a deeper understanding of that information. That means increasing the breadth of research, finding new sources of information, and discovering new ways to interpret it.

I used to think of information as something I found in a book or on a website. As a child, I remember rifling through *Encyclopedia Britannica*, picking up information about everything from astronomy to zoology. But now, I realize that information takes many forms other than words on a page. And I have Mr. Harris to thank for this.

Mr. Harris was a seventy-six-year-old gentleman who had come to the ED because of constipation causing severe pain. This was during one of my rare less-hectic months in residency, when I took time to come into the ED for a couple hours a day "off duty" and simply interact with patients, to see their side of the experience.

After one of my colleagues had completed Mr. Harris's initial history and physical exam, I entered his room and introduced myself. It took a couple minutes to explain that yes, I was a physician, but no, I wasn't *his* physician in this particular case. That I just wanted to sit and talk with him. The reason it took a few minutes to explain was due to Mr. Harris not quite believing me. He was sure I was there to do something, like draw blood or ask more questions about his condition. I assured him I just wanted to talk, if he felt like talking, and offered to leave if he preferred. He then insisted that I stay.

The two-minute patient interaction we had just completed was already different from any other in my seven years of medical training. There was so much packed into those two minutes. My ignorance of the patient's perspective was overwhelming, even after seven years of interacting with them. Across the nation, tens of thousands of residents see patients every day, but hardly any experience the encounter through the patient's eyes.

Mr. Harris's initial confusion in response to my request was telling. He didn't expect to have a conversation. He resisted it reflexively, even suspiciously. He expected business-like efficiency, nothing more. In those initial two minutes of what would turn out to be a two-hour conversation, I experienced just how damaged the relationship between patient and physician has become. And I realized that whatever medical care we are able to deliver is being squeezed through a bottlenecked physician-patient relationship.

I sat down in a chair next to Mr. Harris. I had already learned so much from him. No words came to me. In that silence was the pain of every patient who felt that the physician doesn't really care and can't or won't spend enough time at his or her bedside. In that silence lay the restrictive rules and regulations that keep medical care locked into the ruthless ticking of administrative clocks. In that silence echoed the sadness from which I, as a young physician, was shielding myself.

It overpowered me. I felt like I was hearing silence for the first time in a hospital. It was as if every beep, every alarm, every ring, and every conversation had shut off. I could hear Mr. Harris breathing, the cadence of his inhalations and exhalations giving shape and character to the silence. This time was open for Mr. Harris and his experience. It was not for me to speak the next word or steer the conversation. I had already done that thousands of times.

In those moments, I recognized something. Silence, too, can be information. That silence was conveying something to me about medical care, patients, and myself that I hadn't learned in any standard training. The emotions I felt were also information. They conveyed something subtler than words and concepts.

Information that wasn't available in textbooks was coming to me in different forms. I recognized the information previously hidden in all that was happening around me—the tapping of a foot, the humming of a tune, and the cry of a child. All these were information as much as they were events. I saw that the Big Data movement is only the tip of the iceberg; that once we learn to be aware of the subtler end of the spectrum of experience, Big Data will pale in comparison to what we all can know.

Then Mr. Harris spoke. "I haven't been feeling too good." More silence. "My grandkids were with me a few days ago." The pauses became shorter and more infrequent. "I wish I got to spend more time with them."

Had I been taking a history, I would have quickly brought the conversation back to the "not feeling good" part. But I was free of agendas, and it felt great. Mr. Harris was allowing me to get to know him. I felt he was testing me, releasing information in short bursts like a sputtering faucet. I didn't move an inch in my chair.

After about ten minutes, he was sure that I was intent on staying for the entire conversation. The dam broke and the words poured forth, sentence after sentence, topic after topic, minute after minute. Volumes of information that had been stored as thoughts, memories, emotions, and desires were released. He talked about grandchildren, Vietnam, retirement, loneliness, chronic medical problems, and his dreams. That information had been waiting a long time, in some cases decades, to reach someone else's ears. He now had the chance to say what was true for him.

His face came alive. He morphed into a storyteller with vivid gestures and dramatic facial expressions. I saw his own sense of well-being, a sense that had been in him all along, start to shine forth. I recognized that this experience he was having was as important to his healing as the physical problem from which he suffered.

I would have a similar experience many years later in the ED. A man in his forties had come in because he was feeling suicidal. He was on the verge of tears, struggling to hold them in. I recognized the information expressed in his slouching posture, his worn facial expression, and his downward gaze. He started telling me about his difficulties at home. Tears streamed down his face. I listened.

Six minutes went by and the patient was still talking, uninterrupted. Six minutes may not seem like a long time, but in a busy ED in which you're being pulled every which way, six uninterrupted minutes with anyone is to be cherished. I decided at that point that unless I was pulled away to attend to some impending crisis, I would not interrupt this patient. I recognized that everything about me was sending information to my patient, including the empathy I felt. Information is more than words, more than body language.

A few more minutes passed. My patient continued to share his story. After eleven minutes of nonstop talking, he looked up at me and smiled through his tears. "Thanks, doc." I hadn't said a word.

The entire world around us is influenced and sustained by information. From time immemorial, the various healing systems of the world have reminded us to pay attention to our food, our thoughts, our feelings, and our environment because they understand that everything is *information*, not just figuratively but literally. They understand the ability our experiences have to *in-form*, or shape into form, our well-being.

Light is information. Seasonal affective disorder (SAD) is an example of light directly informing mood. (SAD can also be treated with a particular type of light.) Flashing lights can induce seizures in some patients with epilepsy—another example of information transmission through light.

Sound, too, is information. Look no further than how a love ballad can inform the recollection of a particular tender moment from years past. Scent, taste, texture, thought, emotion, food, social signals—all of these are conveyors of information and therefore influence our well-being.

When the information pouring into our Three Bodies from all sides is not recognized and acted upon, we become passive receivers of their influence and our well-being is compromised. Think about how many times you "just didn't feel right" in a situation. You may not have been in any imminent danger, but your body may have been sending you a signal to either change something in your environment or remove yourself from that environment based on information that was receiving.

Many times, the subtle changes we experience during the course of a day—a mild headache, irritability, calmness, unusual hunger—are due to environmental factors informing our Three Bodies. Because we generally don't subscribe to the idea that we are interconnected with our environment in every moment, such symptoms and relationships often go unrecognized.

This is one way in which unforeseen medical problems arise. They do not begin suddenly. They develop slowly, immersed in and shaped by a sea of information. From this perspective, it is highly inefficient to focus on treating disease with a single pill or procedure. By learning to recognize, respond to, and modify the information all around and within us, we can create a blueprint for our own bodies that restores and sustains well-being.

Over twenty-five years ago, David Bohm, a pioneering theoretical physicist, proposed a model of the universe in which information played the pivotal role. He wrote:

> *This means that that which we experience as mind, in its movement through various levels of subtlety, will, in a natural way ultimately move the body by reaching the level of the quantum potential and of the "dance" of the particles. There is no unbridgeable gap or barrier between any of these levels. Rather, at each stage some kind of information is the bridge.... And through the activity of this information, [mind] similarly takes part in the whole and in every part.... Thus, there is no real division between mind and matter, psyche and soma....*[1]

Bohm's words, and our own investigation of the human body, leave us with three points to reconcile and integrate:

1) Information is a link between subjective and objective experience.
2) There are two categories of energy—subjective (putative) and objective (veritable).
3) Both energy and information are ubiquitous.

Let's dive into these three points and see how we can integrate them:

By acknowledging the ubiquity of energy and information, we can also infer that they must be strongly related. Wherever one is found, the other is found. Thus, both putative and veritable energy must be strongly related to information.

Whereas the information in veritable energy can be measured, the information in putative energy remains so far undecipherable by objective methods. It has remained undecipherable because it is encoded in subjective experience, or mind, whereas the information in veritable energy is encoded in matter. We can use Bohm's understanding of information to bridge these two branches of energy and complete our understanding of it.

Bohm used the concept of information in the broadest sense—as that which *in-forms* or gives form. He writes, "The basic idea of active information is that a form having very little energy enters into and directs a much greater energy. The activity of the latter is in this way given a form similar to that of the smaller energy. It is therefore clear that the original energy-form will "inform" (i.e. put form into) the activity of the larger energy."[2]

With this passage, Bohm draws an important relationship between information and energy by noting that information is itself a form of energy. If we strip away the units that limit energy to a particular dimension or category (i.e., joules, kilowatt-hours), energy is simply *activity*. In relation to information, energy is the activity of information.

Your Physical Body is an energetic formation that has assumed the particular molecular structure of a human body. How does that energy maintain its structure? Why doesn't your body collapse into a heap of atoms or spontaneously reconfigure itself into a pineapple? It's because its energetic structure is an *active* informational structure. *Information* tells the body what configuration to maintain, and *activity* maintains the configuration.

We usually recognize the informational structure at the physical level. The particles that make up your Physical Body, the space between those particles, and the forces that hold them together all have specific properties. Those properties, informing trillions upon trillions of particles, comprise a staggering library of *in-formation* that *forms* your Physical Body.

Furthermore, the information in your Physical Body is not passive. It doesn't sit on the table like a recipe. It self-organizes into your Physical Body. It is therefore *active* information. Information specifies the form; the activity of energy assembles it. Another way of saying this is that

MICHELANGELO'S MEDICINE

information is a specific pattern, while energy is the activity of patterning. The two are inseparable.

In the case of kinetic energy, three variables inform the work—mass, distance, and time. Each of the three variables is a form of information. For example, the fact that an object has a mass of ten kilograms is information that is essential to its kinetic energy. Distance and time also are information informing the object's kinetic energy. Therefore, information is essential to energy.

We further know that passive information will not suffice. The *activity* of that information is what transforms it into energy. After all, the importance of energy is that it has the potential to *do something*. It is this active factor that is shaped by information. In the case of kinetic energy, activity is captured in the movement implied in the relationship of distance per unit time. Taken together, activity and information yield an understanding of energy as *active information*.

Energy as active information applies just as well to potential energy. The information in potential energy takes the form of mass, height, and gravity. The activity is contained in the acceleration of gravity in meters per second squared.

To take another example, a common unit of energy is the joule, which can be simplified to units of kilograms, meters, and seconds—information. The activity captured by the joule is recognized in the relationship of meters squared per second squared: joule = kilograms x $meters^2/seconds^2$

These examples suggest that the common scientific understanding of energy in its objective form fits the definition of active information. This also means that what we understand to be objective energy is only a subset of what energy truly is.

The units we apply to energy, such as joules, capture only the physical dimension of energy, given that joules are merely a combination of kilograms, meters, and seconds. How can we account for the remaining energy that has remained elusive—putative energy? This is where the value of defining energy as active information is truly realized.

If a healer's subjective experience of putative energy correlates strongly with clinical improvement in diseased tissue, it follows that the diseased tissue has acquired new *in-formation* detailing a new, healthier configuration. Not only does the tissue receive the information, it *acts* on it by changing its configuration to that of healthier tissue. We can summarize the proceedings by saying that the healer first detects active information in the form of energy, and subsequently the patient's tissue demonstrates the result of that active information.

Therefore, putative energy also meets the definition of energy as active information. By zeroing in on the mechanism by which information is transferred and activated, we will gain a more complete understanding of energy.

In the Mental Body, information and energy take a subtler form than they do in the Physical Body. By measuring neuronal activity in the brain, we can detect only some aspects of the subtler active information carried in the form of emotions, thoughts, desires, and intuition. The subtlety of information corresponds to what we perceive as increasingly subjective experiences.

In the Energetic Body, information and energy converge. What we call information is seen as a specific type of patterning, and energy is seen as the activity of that patterning. Information cannot be separated from its active form, just as the information that shapes your Physical Body cannot be removed without collapsing your Physical Body. The Energetic Body gives us the understanding that *active information* is a redundant phrase. Information is always active, just as energy always has a pattern.

Information has different meanings in different contexts, but it is active in every one of them. In digital form, information may be the zeroes and ones that inform computers. Even these zeroes and ones are not merely data—they are active information about the flow of voltage in the computer. The meaning encoded in that information then activates the next level of interpretation. In text form, information may be the words and sentences you are reading on this page. These sentences then actively give shape to your own interpretations. Even if you weren't reading these words, they carry the activity of my own thought process. Furthermore, the ink or pixels that form these words are structures made of active particles and energy. Any way you look at it, where there is information, there is activity. Separating the active component is simply a way to conceptualize particular aspects of the unity that is energy and information.

From the above analysis, we can draw three conclusions:

1. Energy and information are aspects of each other.
2. All experiences, subjective and objective, are patterns of energy and information.
3. The Three Bodies are patterns of energy and information.

Today's medical science pays attention to one-third of the human being—the personal Physical Body—because it has an incomplete understanding of energy and information. The result is an incomplete approach to well-being that can perpetuate disease by treating symptoms in the personal Physical Body while leaving the root of disease growing silently in the Energetic and Mental Bodies.

The best of example of this happening is the treatment of one of the most common illnesses there is—an upper respiratory infection, or simply the common cold. If cold symptoms are troubling enough, treatment will often consist of taking pills to alleviate nasal congestion, suppress the cough, and suppress a low-grade fever. Often, the symptoms will improve with this treatment, and over the course of a week or so the immune system will dispose of the offending virus and the patient will get back to a baseline level of health.

What gets missed in the whole rigmarole is the perspective that many people were exposed to the same culprit virus, but only one of them got sick. Furthermore, the person who got sick may have also been going through a highly stressful stretch at work and not sleeping well for the prior week. Stress in the Mental Body then expressed itself at the level of the Physical Body as the symptoms of a common cold. But there's more to the story. What can remain unrecognized is that the Mental Body itself is often left untreated and later expresses as a different illness, perhaps a skin infection or chest pain.

Just as water can transform from vapor to liquid to solid ice, all the while remaining as H_2O, information and energy flow from the Energetic to the Mental to the Physical Body. The mind and body appear to be different only because we focus on their outward appearance. When we shift our attention to see what they are constructed from, they merge into a single process that flows as Three Bodies. The vision of distinct anatomy and physiology is integrated into the vision of a ceaseless stream of energy and information.

The new understanding of the human being as Three Bodies sustained by information and energy has its foundation in established philosophy and science. Philosophically, the outdated, present-day model of human anatomy is based on Cartesian dualism. *Cartesian* refers to its originator, Rene Descartes, and *dualism* refers to the way his philosophy splits human experience into two parts, mind and body. In this instance, mind is what we experience subjectively (happiness, for example) and body is what we see objectively (the smile on a face). Medical science decided long ago that it would cleave subjective experience from objective experience and focus primarily on the latter.

The philosophical systems of idealism and non-dualism take a different approach. They state that all experience is mental. Even our "physical" bodies and the "physical" furniture around us are mental experiences we are having, just as the seemingly-physical objects in a dream are in fact mental experiences. We will explore this in detail in the next chapter.

Idealism and non-dualism are supported by experiments in quantum physics. Once we reach the submicroscopic, quantum realm, the apparent solidness of objects disappears into a world of waves and fields. What we interpret as solid particles is just that—a mental interpretation.

> *Isolated material particles are abstractions, their properties being definable and observable only through their interaction with other systems.*[3]
> —NIELS BOHR, WINNER OF THE 1922 NOBEL PRIZE IN PHYSICS

> *To put the conclusion crudely—the stuff of the world is mind-stuff.*[4]
> — SIR ARTHUR EDDINGTON, ASTROPHYSICIST

This knowledge has not yet saturated the rest of science, especially the medical sciences, including biochemistry, anatomy, physiology, and pathology. The seemingly mysterious, nonphysical quantum world has been walled off from the macroscopic, "solid" world we perceive because most physicists have been unable to reconcile the coexistence of these apparently different worlds. That reconciliation can be facilitated by an intuitive appreciation of the bridge connecting mental and physical experiences.

The scene you are part of right now can be experienced as a scene made up of several objects (including your physical body), a scene comprised of thoughts, or a scene reverberating as energy itself. Without insight from these experiences, it is difficult to place the stepping stones needed to theoretically bridge the quantum (mental) and classical (physical) worlds.

Experiential knowledge begins with regular introspective practice. To capture this knowledge scientifically, we must look more deeply into the nature of energy and information (as outlined above), research how they bridge the experiences of mind and matter, and apply that understanding to current interpretations of quantum mechanics. Then, the personal experience and scientific conclusions we gain must be accommodated within a logically consistent philosophical framework.

Experience, experimentation, and logic must go hand in hand. That doesn't happen today because our experience is focused primarily in the physical and mental bodies, our science is rooted in the outdated philosophy of dualism, and as a result, our logic cannot penetrate the inner workings of mind and matter. This is why we need a Science of Well-Being.

A Science of Well-Being will be rooted in the philosophical perspectives of non-dualism and idealism. It will be logically rigorous, experimentally sound, and just as importantly, intuitive and experienceable. The application of such a science in the field of medicine will be revolutionary. It will be able to translate concepts of energy and information across The Three Bodies, as well as across multiple healing systems.

The field of medicine that is most ready to benefit from a Science of Well-Being is integrative medicine. By establishing a model of interprofessional practice in which each healing system is valued, integrative medicine has demonstrated how different sets of information can coexist complementarily in the same clinical setting. A unifying Science of Well-Being supporting those sets of information has not yet been codified because we haven't yet discovered their common origin. A focus on energy and information will lead us to this convergence point. Integrative medicine is in an ideal position to preserve the deep knowledge within each healing system while also unleashing the power that will come with a unified scientific understanding.

Thousands of years ago, ancient systems such as yoga discovered how to manage The Three Bodies and develop inner technologies to unleash the power inherent in the human being. We are finally approaching the entrance of this information mine. Research into the subtler aspects of human anatomy, such as the body's electromagnetic fields and light production in the form of biophotons, are emerging data points in a Science of Well-Being that will describe the complete human being and establish basic anatomical and physiological principles that are universal, building bridges connecting all healing systems. This isn't science fiction, but rather science nonfiction, and it's happening today in laboratories around the world. It's time for our grade schools, universities, graduate schools, and professional schools to catch up. Our youngest minds must have access to the latest knowledge so that they may unleash its full potential as they grow.

Here are the characteristics of the emerging Science of Well-Being:

- It recognizes the potential inherent in every human being.
- It recognizes all matter as informational and energetic in nature.
- It bridges mind and matter through a more complete understanding of information and energy.
- It provides a theoretical foundation for integrative medicine and personal well-being.
- It provides a link between the emerging understanding of the human biofield and allopathic science.
- It amplifies the healing potential of bioinformatics, the digital revolution in medical care, genomics, and precision medicine, by providing a complete model of the informational and energetic human being.

Here, then, is the evolutionary life cycle of the aggregate healing system of the world—presented in order from past to future:

1) Various <u>healing systems</u> emphasize the importance of the human being's relationship with nature and the environment. <u>Healing systems</u> are unique to specific populations, their values, and their circumstances.
2) The human organism and its parts are dissected from its greater environment so that ever-smaller aspects of the organism can be studied. This is the reductionist movement.
3) Allopathic medicine reaches its peak as a stand-alone <u>healing system,</u> and medical treatment comes to be defined by its successes in treating acute illness and deficiencies in treating chronic illness. Other <u>healing systems</u> are collectively termed *alternative medicine.*
4) New explorations combine ancient and modern principles to find balance in medical care. <u>Integrative medicine</u> emerges as the standard-bearer of a true <u>health care system,</u> based on an interprofessional model that values the unique approach of each <u>healing system</u>. The clinical success of <u>integrative medicine</u> further spurs the development of a Science of Well-Being.
5) Information and energy form the basis of a Science of Well-Being, bridging our experience and understanding of mind and matter. Our understanding of human anatomy evolves from the Physical Body to the mind-body to <u>The Three Bodies</u>. The unique approach of each <u>healing system</u> becomes available to all. A Science of Well-Being informs the development of safe, accessible, effective, and powerful innate and external technologies that optimize well-being and heal the whole human being.

Key Points

- Information and energy are two aspects of the same entity. Information is a specific pattern and energy is the activity of patterning.
- The definition of energy as *active information* can bridge our understanding of putative and veritable energy, and of mind and matter.

- The emerging Science of Well-Being is defined by its comprehensive understanding of the relationship between mind, information, energy, matter, and human anatomy and physiology.
- A Science of Well-Being is validated not only by scientific experimentation but also by personal experience and a sound philosophical basis.
- <u>Integrative medicine</u> is poised to be the standard-bearer of a true <u>health care system</u>, based in a Science of Well-Being.

Q&A

- *Q: What is information?*
  A: Information is a pattern. For example, a ripple in a lake is a pattern of water. It is also a *form* of water. It is in-*form*-ation. The feeling of joy is a pattern of the mind. It is also a *form* of the mind. It, too, is in-*form*-ation. A chair is a pattern of particles and a pattern of energy. It is also a formation of particles and of energy. The chair is in-*form*-ation.
- *Q: What is energy?*
  A: Energy is the activity of a pattern—the pattern-*ing* that sustains the pattern. A ripple in a lake is also a *rippling*—an activity. That activity is energy. The feeling of joy is an activity of the mind. That activity is energy. A chair is sustained by the constant activity of particles. That activity is energy.
- *Q: How will a Science of Well-Being bridge mind and matter?*
  A: The concepts of information and energy give us a way to bridge the activity we subjectively recognize in the mind with activity we can objectively note as matter. This is the foundation of a Science of Well-Being. The feeling of wanting to go outside on a sunny day is subjective information. That feeling may become the thought "I'm going to go for a walk"—subjective information that now may also be recordable with neuroimaging; it is becoming objective. That thought then becomes the physical action of stepping outside, which now carries information that is distinctly objective and recordable. At each step along the way, information—and therefore energy—plays a central role.

- *Q: Why do we need a Science of Well-Being?*
  A: Today's medical science sees only one-third of the human being—the personal Physical Body. The result is an incomplete approach to well-being that can perpetuate disease. A Science of Well-Being will provide a logical, experiential, and experimentally verified model of entire human being and will establish basic anatomical and physiological principles that are universal, providing a bridge between all healing systems.
- *Q: Will integrative medicine dilute the knowledge of individual healing systems?*
  A: No. Integrative medicine is comprised of the information contained in all healing systems. While it can cross-reference among different approaches to healing, it doesn't replace the unique knowledge within each one.

References

1. David Bohm, "A New Theory of the Relationship of Mind and Matter," *Philosophical Psychology* 3:2, 271–86.
2. Bohm, D., & Hiley, B. J. (2005). The undivided universe: An ontological interpretation of quantum theory. London: Routledge.
3. Bohr, Niels (1934). Atomic Theory and the Description of Nature. Ox Bow Press.
4. Eddington, Arthur Stanley (1928). The Nature of the Physical World.

CHAPTER 13
What is the Next Step in the Evolution of Science?

The Informational Problem is not unique to medical science. It applies to all of science. Just as the body is not only a physical structure but also an energetic one, all experiences are energetic in nature, including thoughts, feelings, and desires.

We have not scientifically appreciated this so far because <u>normal science</u> (a term coined by Thomas Kuhn in his seminal work *The Structure of Scientific Revolutions*) learns about the world by objectifying it. Energy cannot be known in its entirety by <u>normal science</u> because energy is equal parts subjective and objective, as experienced by the human being.

Despite lacking this understanding, <u>normal science</u> has succeeded brilliantly in solving many problems, including the treatment of acute, life-threatening illness in many cases. Outside of medical care, I am still amazed every time I look out the window of a plane as it takes off—a seventy-ton behemoth behaving as though it's lighter than a feather.

As marvelous as the achievements of <u>normal science</u> are, we should not fail to ask what its fundamental limitations are and what we can do to address them. The success of <u>normal science</u> is a testament to our creativity and intelligence as a species, not a final validation of the way it has interpreted the world.

An objective model of the world has been useful for us to describe the universe from the atomic to the cosmic scale, but it cannot take us the distance because science is ultimately a human endeavor and therefore necessarily subjective. It is naturally influenced by personal bias and the boundaries of human perception and thinking. The universe itself has no such boundaries. Human limitations of perception have gotten us in trouble before. We thought for a long time that the sun revolved around the Earth, and propagated that idea, supported by science. But, in fact, it was a myth.

> *If these out-of-date beliefs are to be called myths, then myths can be produced by the same sorts of methods and held for the same sorts of reasons that now lead to scientific knowledge.*[1]
> —Thomas Kuhn

The biggest myth in science today is that we can know enough about the world by studying it objectively. Suppose I wander off course on a safari and meet with the rare opportunity of seeing an okapi up close. (An okapi, as I recently learned from my son, is an animal that has the striped legs of a zebra and the trunk, neck, and head of a giraffe. Yes, it's a real animal.)

According to normal science, what I am seeing is not an okapi, but rather a construction of my brain. The story goes that before I ever see the animal, photons ricochet off the would-be okapi in front of me, strike my retina, send a signal to my brain, and are then interpreted into the image of an okapi in my brain. That image is then projected as though it's in the field in front of me. *Only then* do I "see" an okapi.

In other words, the okapi doesn't exist *out there*. The image is inherently subjective and dependent on the type of nervous system that interprets it. A bat's nervous system uses echolocation to "see" at night. It doesn't see our version of the okapi. There are as many interpretations of an okapi as there are species on Earth, leaving aside members of the same species with different perspectives. Which is the "real" reality?

What we call objective reality is actually a subjective interpretation. The very room around you is a subjective interpretation of your brain and nervous system, as is your own body. There is no independent, external reality. But it gets even more radical than that.

There is a critical limitation in what I just explained: It already assumes a "real brain" that interprets the image of an okapi, whereas, in fact, the brain is itself a subjective interpretation. Once upon a time, anatomists opened the skull, saw the brain, and drew connections between the brain and the body's functions, and today the brain is known as the control center of the body. Nothing about this story implies that the brain is intrinsically more real than the world it interprets. On the contrary, the brain itself is a mental interpretation of anatomists, and continues to be a mental interpretation we (usefully) make today. The brain, the body, and the rest of the world are mental experiences. In other words, the brain and body are in the mind, not the other way around.

Normal science believes in and depends on the perception of an *external* world independent of us because its unexamined assumptions about the nature of the world leave it no recourse. It leans on perception, but doesn't completely understand it. It is steeped in a tradition that believes the world around us is a jigsaw puzzle that can be solved by studying each piece independent of ourselves, failing to see that we are shaping the pieces as we study them.

> *Under normal conditions the research scientist is not an innovator but a solver of puzzles, and the puzzles upon which he concentrates are just those which he believes can be both stated and solved within the existing scientific tradition.*[1]
> —THOMAS KUHN

Today, we can't logically explain how we smell warm apple pie. The best explanation we have is that an electrical firing in the brain is associated with the smell of pie, which is almost like no explanation at all. An electrical signal does not resemble the smell of apple pie in any way—they are simply in different ballparks. So how does the experience of scent actually arise? How does *any* experience arise?

If we can't answer a question this fundamental, how much can we really claim to know about how the body and mind work? How much can we claim to know about subtleties like well-being, healing, and illness?

The failure of normal science to recognize that we are shaping the world and our understanding of it by the very methods we use to study it has created a ceiling to our understanding, a very real barrier to knowledge. Therefore, the domain beyond that ceiling is generally restricted to philosophy, spirituality, and religion.

In fact, all of these human endeavors, including science, are not so different. They all represent the human being's thirst to know about the universe and our relationship with it. All of them—some below and some above the ceiling of objective knowledge—can be accommodated across a single continuum of understanding.

Below the ceiling, subjective and objective knowledge appear separate, even independent of each other. This is the domain of <u>normal science</u>. As the ceiling is approached, subjective experience appears to influence objective phenomena, the most popular example of which is that simply measuring activity at the quantum scale appears to influence the behavior of particles and waves.

Above the ceiling, objective phenomena are seen as a subset of subjective experience, insofar as anything that can be known must be within our experience. Subjective experience is as fundamental as objective measurements. This is the second domain of understanding, which has its own ceiling. Beyond that second ceiling, subjective and objective perspectives converge.

> *The world of duality, which is perceived to exist and is characterized by the subject-object relationship, is a movement of the mind.* [2]
> —Gaudapada, ~AD 600

> *I consider those developments in physics during the last decades which have shown how problematical such concepts as "objective" and "subjective" are, a great liberation of thought.* [3]
> —Niels Bohr, winner of the 1922 Nobel Prize in Physics

This continuum of understanding bridges <u>normal science</u>, philosophy, spirituality, and religion. What remains to be done is to clarify the nature of the ceiling we are bumping against with a more complete understanding of <u>information</u> and <u>energy</u>. This will require not just objective experimentation but subjective exploration of our own inner experience.

The great scientists of tomorrow will adventure not just outwardly through microscopes and telescopes but also inwardly, turning the observing lens on their own minds. Such an approach will lead to insights that complete the bridge between consciousness and matter, mind and body, and subjective and objective experience.

I've often heard the comment that science isn't about metaphysics. Some say we should leave normal science alone. Yet the very science we practice today is already metaphysical. Science is a cyclical process of making observations, forming hypotheses, and conducting experiments. To state the obvious, each aspect—observing, hypothesizing, and experimenting—is occurring in the minds of scientists, not in a conjured objective reality. Furthermore, normal science has assumed a dualistic philosophical stance. It is soaked in metaphysical assumptions already. It's time we understand their implications.

Another comment I've heard is that we are doing well enough already. Normal science has solved many great problems, so the story goes that we should expect it to solve the rest of them, too, including explaining how something like the flux of ions in a neuron yields the experience of falling in love. But the answer to this basic problem—and to the problem of how we have any experience at all—doesn't fall within the current scientific paradigm. The answer is patiently waiting above the ceiling, watching for signs of normal science's arrival.

If we are to call ourselves a modern scientific society, we must embrace these facts instead of run from them. Indeed, we have started to embrace them already. Some scientists are daring to break through the ceiling. They are accounting for the holes in normal science by moving the mind toward the center of the puzzle.

> *All that we see, we project out of our own minds.*[4]
> —SWAMI VIVEKANANDA

> *That is to say, I think our consciousness is not just a passive epiphenomenon carried along by the chemical events in our brains, but is an active agent forcing the molecular complexes to make choices between one quantum state and another. In other words, mind is already inherent in every electron....*[5]
> —FREEMAN DYSON, THEORETICAL PHYSICIST

What is this *consciousness* that physicists, philosophers, and sages are talking about?

Our consciousness is the one thing that we cannot logically deny. Before we classify experiences as subjective or objective, before we interpret science and ceilings, and before we feel happy or sad, we must be conscious. Without consciousness, there is no experience whatsoever. It is the primal factor that makes any and all experience possible.

Consciousness is an abstract word used in many ways. We could talk about the state of waking consciousness (which I'm in as I write this), dream consciousness, pre-consciousness, sub-consciousness, and so on. We could also talk about human consciousness and animal consciousness. But what I am referring to by using the word *consciousness* in this context is something more fundamental than all of these subtypes: Consciousness is that which gives rise to any and all experience, including the experience of "me," of science, and of an apparently physical world.

> *Consciousness cannot be accounted for in physical terms. For consciousness is absolutely fundamental. It cannot be accounted for in terms of anything else.*[6]
> — ERWIN SCHRODINGER, NOBEL PRIZE-WINNING PHYSICIST

We can trace a path to consciousness by recalling the role of information and energy as a bridge between mind and matter. What we refer to as information is a pattern of some kind. That pattern must be a pattern *of something*. A pattern on a shirt is made of thread and dye. A pattern drawn on paper is made of graphite from the tip of a pencil. In the case of information itself, that pattern is a pattern of consciousness.

We saw in the last chapter that energy can be understood as active information. More fundamentally, we can see that if information itself is a pattern of consciousness, then energy is the activity of consciousness. In other words, information is a way of describing specific patterns in consciousness, and energy is a way of describing activities of consciousness. Since every pattern is also an activity and every activity has some pattern, information and energy are not fundamentally different. They are facets of each other: information-energy.

consciousness <—information-energy—> **mind** <—information-energy—> **matter**

What is the nature of consciousness? Is it happy? Joyful? Irritated? Restless? (After all, it has the gall to display quite the array of experiences.) Remember that what we are referring to as consciousness here is not a subtype such as human or animal consciousness, which are patterns within undifferentiated consciousness. Undifferentiated or unpatterned consciousness cannot be accurately captured in words because words are themselves patterns.

> *The Tao that can be spoken is not the eternal Tao.*[7]
> —Lao Tzu

Language and thinking can capture only aspects of consciousness, or patterns of it, such as "science," or "matter." Nevertheless, let's attempt the impossible and describe consciousness, having noted the inherent limitations.

Existence is the nature of consciousness. Consciousness has to exist for any of our experiences to exist. That existence must also be *aware*. If not, how could awareness arise in the mind? Awareness must be of the intrinsic nature of existence for it to become apparent down the line.

Finally, that *existence-awareness* must also be *limitless* because it gives rise to any and all experience, including the experience of space and time. The nature of consciousness can therefore be said to be *existence-awareness-limitlessness*, or more palatably, *awareness without boundaries*. It is important to remember that this description is not of human consciousness, which does have boundaries because it is a particular pattern of consciousness. However, this consciousness is available to everyone through introspection and unpatterning the mind.

Many other cultures around the world have their own descriptions of the fundamental factor at the heart of existence. Whatever its name and description, what it *is* cannot differ among cultures, sciences, and traditions. Only interpretations can differ.

> *I regard consciousness as fundamental. I regard matter as derivative from consciousness. We cannot get behind consciousness. Everything that we talk about, everything that we regard as existing, postulates consciousness.*[8]
> — MAX PLANCK, 1931, NOBEL PRIZE-WINNING PHYSICIST

The Three Bodies are patterns of consciousness, or information-energy, expressing as an Energetic Body, a Mental Body, and a Physical Body. These Three Bodies are what we call "me," the individual human being. By turning inward, we can trace our path back to unpatterned consciousness, or *being* — the masterpiece at the heart of well-*being*. To do so is to experience your fullness beyond The Three Bodies, beyond individuality, beyond any sense of separateness. This is not a religious, spiritual, philosophical, or scientific inquiry. It is simply practical.

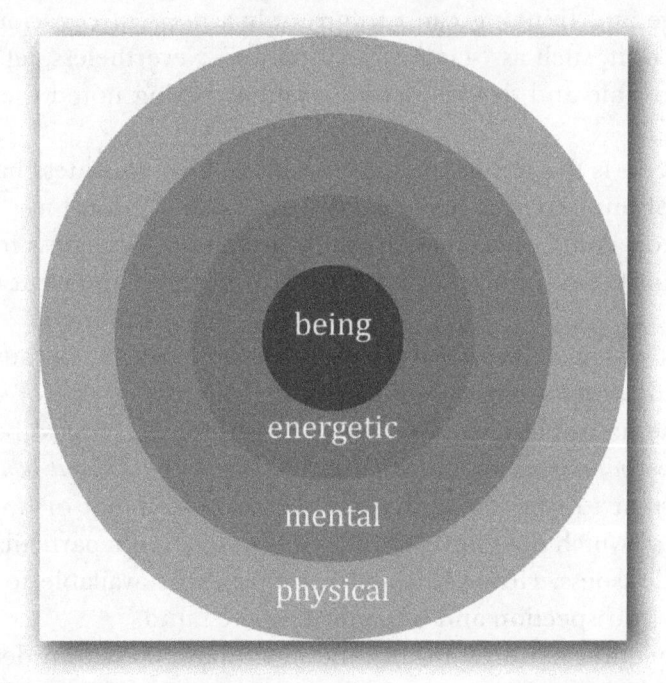

Consciousness touches each one of us. It is alive and palpable within us. It is as available and relevant to a child as it is to an adult, to the poor as it is to the rich, and to the ill as it is to the well. Consciousness does not discriminate on any basis because the very notion of *difference* doesn't exist within it. Most importantly, it is practical, because a lack of appreciation of the consciousness within us distorts and magnifies the apparent differences among us—the leading cause of the biggest problems we face today. When we see differences more clearly than similarity, we fight over resources instead of cooperating to innovate beyond scarcity.

When I look out at the scene in front of me, I see a laptop, a wall, a carpet, and some furniture. Each of these objects has one thing in common: it is finite. When I appreciate the laptop as simply an object in front of me, I can assign it a weight, a shape, and a color. In other words, I can mentally reduce it to a series of finite measurements.

Anything that is finite can become scarce at any moment. If my laptop stops working, I have to scramble for another one. If my car runs out of gas, I seek out the closest gas station. Even something as massive as the Earth is also scarce. There's only one Earth, after all.

When I see something external to me (like this laptop I'm typing on), I am recognizing only a part of it. To see the whole picture, I also have to see what is common to both me and the laptop—unpatterned consciousness, which is expressing as this scene I'm a part of. This has to ultimately be done not just analytically, not just scientifically, but directly, unmediated by thought. Slipping behind the brain's staging of the events is necessary in order to see through the mental conditioning that suggests that I am something separate and independent from everything around me.

When attention shifts from the object *out there* to the consciousness that is *here*, the experience of separation ends. This is the gateway to unpatterned consciousness. This is the gateway out of a scarcity paradigm and into an abundance paradigm.

In unpatterned consciousness, abundance is standard and innovation is the norm because we are tapping into pure potential. Innovation is the antidote for scarcity. For example, energy is scarce if we are thinking only about fossil fuels. If we harness other forms of energy, energy becomes abundant. In isolation, love seems scarce. But if attention is shifted away from self-limiting thoughts and toward our innate consciousness, love is found in abundance. There is nothing more practical than this.

Scientists bold enough to step outside the assumptions of <u>normal science</u> are beginning to acknowledge the central role of consciousness in our understanding of the universe, as evidenced by the growing number of papers and books on the topic. As you read this, researchers around the world are developing a science of consciousness (a key part of a Science of Well-Being) that embraces and accounts for subjective and objective aspects of experience. Such a science goes by many names, including <u>observer-based science</u>, subjective science, and qualia science.

An observer-based science begins with the understanding that the universe is recognized and experienced only in consciousness. Therefore, consciousness and the universe cannot be separated, except as a concept. Secondly, everything that we know about this universe is known as an experience that we are having. Therefore, this science also recognizes that experiences can be thought of as discrete units of consciousness—fundamental patterns—and therefore they are the building blocks of the universe we perceive. This replaces the objective scientific notion that the universe is made of particles, waves, fields, and space.

Every experience you have, whether of enjoying ice cream, being in a heated argument, or drifting off to sleep, is a distinct pattern within the greater unpatterned consciousness. Unpatterned consciousness is generally forgotten because specific patterns are so compelling and attention-grabbing, that is, the ice cream is so tasty, the argument is so personal, the sleep is so welcoming. Such experiences, or patterns, are the very building blocks of the universe.

Once upon a time, we used to think atoms were the building blocks of the universe. The very word *atom* means not-cut, or indivisible. But we discovered later that the atom is divisible into subatomic and elementary particles. No matter how small a particle we discover, we can trace it further back to a wave, a field, and even further into seeming nothingness. But no matter how far we go, there is no getting around the fact that what we discover will still be an *experience* that we are having in the mind, suggesting that space, time, and mind are convergent concepts.

We can say that experience is the building block of the universe because a complete experience includes both subjective and objective aspects. Any experience, such as that of eating an orange, includes the experiencer (the person/subject eating the orange) and whatever it is that he or she is experiencing (the object), in this case the orange. Therefore, considering experience as a whole bridges subjective and objective reality, which can take us beyond the ceiling of objective understanding.

Extracting experience as a unit of consciousness, and therefore as the building block of the universe, allows us to plug and play the objective science we have developed over hundreds of years within the context of a modern, observer-based science. Observer-based science first provides the framework for the subjective and objective aspects of the unit of experience. Then, objective science further fills in the objective aspect of the unit of experience.

A more complete understanding of information and energy will lead to the recognition that information and energy are aspects of each other (an active pattern and a pattern of activity). We will then be able to discern that they are present both in the subject and in the object through the following line of questioning.

In the example above, the person eating the orange is one pattern and the orange itself is another pattern. This inevitably will lead to a convergent line of questioning: What are they both a pattern *of?* What is common to both subject and object?

This will also lead to a divergent line of questioning: What is objective experience? How can we differentiate it from subjective experience using the concept of information? The answer is that when we look at the subjective aspect of experience, we can note its qualitative informational components, such as its sights (the spherical appearance and the orange color), sounds (the squishing sound made by biting into the orange), smells, tastes, and textures.

These components, called qualia, can be mapped to a quantified, projected physical reality, which is where today's objective science begins. In the above example, the spherical appearance of the orange may be mapped to a quantified measurement, such as a diameter of six centimeters. The orange color can be mapped to a wavelength of 600 nanometers. The appearance may also be mapped to the activation of a particular part of the occipital cortex of the brain. The squishing sound could be mapped to a particular frequency and duration.

The benefits of such a science are that it doesn't leave out any aspect of human experience; it appreciates and encourages both objective and observer-based approaches, while reconciling the two; it contextualizes the physical universe as a projection in consciousness; it can lead to the development of new technologies; and finally and most importantly, it can free us from a limiting, constricting understanding and experience of ourselves. In short, it is a complete science.

To summarize, we have six principles forming the foundation of an observer-based science:

1) The universe is essentially consciousness itself.
2) Experiences are units of consciousness.
3) The fundamental building blocks of the universe are experiences.
4) Experiences have subjective and objective components that can be understood in terms of information and energy.
5) The objective, physical universe is a quantified subset of information that describes a part of the unit of experience.
6) Today's objective science is the subset of observer-based science that studies quantified, partial projections.
7) A complete science integrates observer-based *and* objective perspectives.

Key Points

- We shape the objects we are observing by the very act of observing them.
- What normal science calls objective reality is an interpretation of the human nervous system. In that sense, it is entirely subjective.
- Reality is beyond subjective and objective perspectives. Reality is not divided by perspectives. Perspectives are aspects of reality.
- Consciousness, or *being*, is the foundation of the universe.
- Consciousness can be described as *limitless awareness*.
- A complete science must account for consciousness, which expresses as subjective and objective perspectives.
- A complete science includes observer-based science and objective science.

- A complete science is founded on the understanding that the universe can be known to exist only in consciousness.

References

1. Kuhn, T. S. (1970). The structure of scientific revolutions. University of Chicago Press.
2. Gaudapada. (~AD 600). Mandukya Karika.
3. Heisenberg, W. (1981). Physics and beyond. London: Allen & Unwin.
4. Vivekananda, S. (1971). The complete works of Swami Vivekananda. Calcutta: Advaita Ashrama.
5. Dyson, F. J. (2001). Disturbing the universe. New York: Basic Books.
6. American Society for Psychical Research. (1931). Psychic Research Volume 25). Fair Lawn, N.J: American Society for Psychical Research.
7. Laozi. Dornberg, C., & Deer's Run Press. (2004). Tao te ching. Tucson, Ariz: Deer's Run Press.
8. As quoted in The Observer (1931)

CHAPTER 14
What will Medical Training Look Like in the Future?

"*I am going to medical school!!!*" Ayesha shrieked and flung her admissions letter up toward the ceiling in delight. It was the culmination of a lifelong dream.

For the past eight years through high school and college, Ayesha had done everything she could to make this day a reality. She couldn't believe it was happening. Wearing a wide grin across her face, she squeezed her parents tightly as their tears brimmed over.

Ayesha gaining entry into medical school had a special significance for her family. Her grandfather, an oncologist by training, had been the last in a long line of physicians in the family. But he abruptly left his lucrative practice relatively early in his career, around the time Ayesha was born. It was something that the family didn't talk about much. Her grandfather dissuaded her father from going to medical school, but Ayesha couldn't be deterred.

The world of medicine that Ayesha was entering was a different world from the one her grandfather trained in. In the years leading up to her medical school admission, Ayesha had already learned much of the first couple years of medical science through free online academies. Information was everywhere, easy to access, free, and customized for an individual's learning experience. The challenge was no longer finding information, but instead determining what information was relevant and reliable.

Ayesha particularly enjoyed holographic learning. The display on her mediaphone projected a hologram of herself into the space in front of her. She could then walk around and into the hologram, asking questions and having it teach her the basics of anatomy and physiology. For example, she could pause frames at each stage of the cardiac cycle to literally see the heart pumping blood throughout the body. She could walk around these frames to see the action from every angle. To learn about histology at the microscopic level, the hologram simply zoomed in to the cellular level.

But it didn't stop there. Beyond the cellular level, the hologram could display the Energetic Body, including the major and minor pathways. It was possible to directly see how the Physical Body was an interpretation, and how energy interfaced with it.

None of this was abstract for Ayesha. The changes in physics, medical science, and health care that had occurred over the last couple decades meant the Physical, Mental, and Energetic Bodies were common, experiential knowledge. Young children intuitively understood these descriptions of their experience. It wasn't "taught out" of them like it was to children just a couple generations before. Children attending school were exposed to the basics of complete human anatomy right from the beginning. It just made sense to learn to recognize what you are while still a child.

When she began her first semester of medical school, Ayesha felt right at home. Anatomy, physiology, histology, and embryology were all describing her as she already knew herself. There were many details and relationships to learn, but the basic framework medical schools around the world were using was based on the complete human experience that every person around the world shared, including physical, intellectual, emotional, and energetic aspects.

Ayesha was collaborating with health practitioners from every <u>healing system</u> around the world right from day one. The Association of American Medical Colleges had declared years before that interdisciplinary education was essential to becoming a competent physician. It was a momentous announcement at the time. They had explained that every physician had to know the strengths and weaknesses of their approach to healing, as well as the strengths and weaknesses of all <u>healing systems</u> so that patients had the best chance possible to heal and experience well-being.

MICHELANGELO'S MEDICINE

Since that announcement, most academic regulatory organizations, representing an array of health practitioners and healing systems, had reciprocated. There was now a free flow of knowledge among all groups.

Ayesha especially enjoyed how different practitioners used their own specific anatomical and physiological terms as they explained their healing system to a class of budding allopaths. Although each practitioner spoke from a different angle, using a different vocabulary, they were all essentially describing aspects of The Three Bodies. The same framework Ayesha had learned as a six-year-old in elementary school was being used in medical school.

What was different was that now she was learning more details and more relationships: how allopathic anatomy interfaced with ayurvedic anatomy; how information and energy appeared as The Three Bodies; how every stimulus was a form of information and energy, and therefore influenced the state of The Three Bodies; how the integration of quantum and classical physics was an intellectual template for the integration of consciousness and matter; how all these equally informed the well-being of both patient and physician; and, of course, how all these influenced the processes of disease and healing. While the information was new, it fit into the same framework she had intuitively learned as a child. It just made sense. Ayesha smiled.

The effect of having a logically rigorous yet intuitive framework for healing and well-being was that the way we viewed intelligence itself had changed. Intellectual knowledge had become a framework for experiential, intuitive understanding rather than an obstacle to it. Medical students were now learning large volumes of information more easily and in a much shorter period of time because they didn't have to fight their intuition; they could experience the information they were learning. Understanding and utilizing emotion was intelligence. Creativity was intelligence. Applicants to medical school were selected based on their aptitude for healing both themselves and future patients, as well as their ability to understand and teach a framework for healing.

Ayesha had begun a practice of meditation when she was ten years old. She found that it helped her to manage herself during stressful times, like when she had several exams coming up. Whenever she felt like she might get off track, she availed herself of a health coach, who was always available for medical students.

Her health coach somehow always knew what would get her back on track. Sometimes it was physical exercise, sometimes taking a couple days off to simply relax or visit family, sometimes simply getting back to her studies. Whatever it was, Ayesha and her health coach had the final say over her academic schedule. If an extra day off were needed, the professors would accommodate it. By being flexible and respecting students' individuality, medical schools were teaching future physicians to do the same for themselves, their patients, and their families.

Medical school came and went quickly for Ayesha. Before she knew it, she had started her family medicine residency at a prestigious program. All the while, her grandfather had said little to her about health care or her career, other than the congratulations he offered when she first learned she had been accepted to medical school.

Residency training hours were long, but manageable enough to allow time for the development of other interests. On especially long shifts, residents availed themselves of chambers that would leave them rejuvenated. These chambers were fitted with light and sound technology that customized therapeutic frequencies for each person. Twenty minutes spent resting in the "sleep shop," as the residents called it, felt like the equivalent of four hours of sleep. Productivity, quality of care, learning, and quality of life benefited greatly.

Halfway through her residency, fresh off giving a presentation on clinical biophysics, Ayesha got a message from her grandfather. He wanted to have lunch. She wasn't sure quite what to expect. Although they had communicated intermittently over the years, she felt a twinge of unease at his request.

Two days later, they met at Ayesha's favorite lunch spot. She wanted to make sure she'd be as comfortable as possible. Her grandfather sat silently, buttering his bread and staring right past her. She knew he was mulling over what he would say. Eventually, he spoke.

"You know, Ayesha, you're lucky." He stared off again. Ayesha thought it best not to interrupt.

"You're lucky." Again, his voice trailed off.

"You're lucky because you're in a system that understands you. It understands that you can't give what you don't have." He took a bite of his bread, paused, and then started to chew slowly.

Ayesha remained quiet. She could feel the emotion with which he was speaking.

He continued, "When I was doing my medical training, resting, eating, and caring for myself in general were the last things on anyone's mind, including my own. But I toughed it out." He swallowed hard.

"In fact, toughing it out become my motto. I later toughed it out during my fellowship, and again toughed it out during my busy clinical practice. Everyone kept telling me how successful I was, but I felt like I was always fighting for something I could never get."

Ayesha offered some words of comfort. "You were a great doctor. Your patients loved you."

"Yeah, most of them did." A weak smile crossed his face. "But medicine shouldn't be about fighting yourself, struggling to make sense of things that don't make sense, or feeling one thing and being taught another. It wears you down. It makes you wonder what you got yourself into."

He wasn't sure Ayesha would even follow what he was saying. Her experience had been so different. Even though he hadn't been talking to her much during her residency, he had been keeping tabs on her progress through her father.

But Ayesha did know what he was talking about. She knew health care had not always been the way it was now. She knew that burnout in health care had been four times the current rate. She knew that clinicians didn't always have enough time with their patients. And she knew that patients and practitioners never really understood themselves the way they did today.

Ayesha walked around the table and gave her grandfather a big hug.

"You're right, Grandpa. I am lucky."

Part III
How we Get There

CHAPTER 15
Dear Clinician

Dear Clinician,

It's obvious that medical care is changing. Sometimes it seems like every day brings another hoop to jump through. What is obvious, yet largely ignored amidst all the mouse clicks and meetings, is that our own well-being impacts the care we give our patients. We, too, are human.

Most of us were trained in programs that gave little consideration to our own well-being. Food was a luxury, or a candy bar—often both. A good night's sleep wasn't in our vocabulary. We've developed a hard-nosed, press-on-at-any-cost approach to medical training and healing that is antithetical to the very phrase *health care.*

If we want to establish a practice that serves our patients best *and* fulfills us, we must lead the change in medical care. We must speak up for our patients, because the well-being of our patients and our own well-being are intertwined.

This brings us face-to-face with an unavoidable question: How can we bring well-being to this system as long as the very science we are taught doesn't understand well-being? We have gotten so used to managing disease and treading water that it's easy to overlook the fact that we do not have a Science of Well-Being but rather a science of disease. Our patients, our profession, and each of us hold ourselves to the highest of standards, yet our science falls short of it. Too often, we succeed *in spite of* medical science's remarkably incomplete understanding of the human being—of you, of me, and of our patients.

We have spent years learning about the human body and disease—reading about it, thinking about it, talking about it, making presentations on it, and (still) taking tests on it. But by dutifully following the track laid by our training, we have been missing out on valuable information about well-being that has been around for millennia—information that is increasingly being confirmed by modern science.

Science is an evolving process, so incompleteness is understandable, but in the medical treatment system, incompleteness harms. We cannot turn a blind eye toward information that has the potential to heal and reduce suffering, no matter where it comes from or how unfamiliar it may appear. We cannot turn a blind eye to the sacred tenet at the heart of our profession—do no harm.

I've made the case in this book that the knowledge we were taught is incomplete, but that doesn't mean it's irrelevant or wrong. I still use it effectively in the ED for my patients, and you can continue to use it for yours. We don't have to retrain ourselves in a new program or read another fifteen textbooks to catch up. We can simply see what we already know in a new light and be open to filling in the blanks from a new perspective.

As the increasing demand for quality in medical care is met by an increasing number of rules and regulations, I predict the clinician's role in championing well-being and healing will become more important than ever. But that will happen only if we inquire into the nature of well-being and healing, and use that fresh knowledge to develop a true health care system.

We are the ones who guide the minds of the next generation of clinicians. We have burned the midnight oil studying for exams for years on end, and we will continue to take exams for the duration of our careers, all the while assuming that we are digesting the latest and best information. Who better to point out the magnitude of the Informational Problem? The responsibility and opportunity are ours. This is the single biggest issue in the medical treatment system today. Our patients are counting on us to stand up for them.

The old paradigm of a machine-like physical body made of ball-and-stick molecules is dying. The more we cling we to it, the more out of touch we become. Patients and clinicians are already too often treated like machines. We unknowingly add fuel to that fire by subscribing to the old paradigm.

The human element of medicine, based in an understanding of well-being and healing, is needed to balance and guide the technological leaps that are being made as you read these words. This is the new paradigm. It is a paradigm in which qualitative experience is known to influence quantitative measurements; a paradigm that encourages the exploration and application of qualitative experience in healing; a paradigm that recognizes the well-being of the clinician cannot be separated from the well-being of the patient; a paradigm that recognizes the value that each healing system can contribute.

If you're like me, you may be thinking, "I'm way too busy to do anything about this. I can barely get my charts done!" I've had the same thoughts, and I don't have all the answers, but I can tell you what works for me.

The first step is to expand your knowledge base online. If you do a search on integrative medicine, for example, you'll find a range of websites. Some extol its miraculous abilities and others vilify it as pseudoscience. As is the case for any controversial topic, there are experts on both sides of the issue. I find that if an expert is exclusionist and can't appreciate what both sides have to contribute, they are likely part of the problem, not the solution. Take the middle path. Scan for information that opens up your perspective on what is possible and take with a grain of salt anything suggesting an effortless panacea for all illness.

The next step is to learn about organizations that are exploring how well-being can be systematized in medical care. This again can be begun online. Here's a list of a few that I've come across.

Academic Consortium for Integrative Medicine and Health, imconsortium.org
Academy of Integrative Health and Medicine, aihm.org
American Holistic Nursing Association, ahna.org
Association for Comprehensive Energy Psychology, energypsych.org
Consciousness and Healing Initiative, chi.is
Integrative Health Policy Consortium, ihpc.org
Integrative Medical Consortium, integrativemedicalconsortium.org
Samueli Institute, samueliinstitute.org

The third and most important step is to start exploring your own mind. More than anything else, this is what will change your understanding of yourself, patient care, and medical science. Consider the possibility that you have been accessing only one part of yourself, and the rest of you is waiting patiently to be discovered.

Refer back to the exercise in the chapter on <u>The Three Bodies</u> and begin a practice of meditation. It can be done in as little as a few seconds—anywhere, anytime. A few easy breaths are all it takes to start.

With these simple steps, your experience of medicine will change surely and steadily. Once you expand your knowledge base, you will never again be able to stuff yourself back into any one perspective on well-being and healing. As your experience continues to broaden, you will experience first-hand what integration and healing mean, and in turn be able to offer it to your patients in any setting.

This is a historic period, not only in medical care but specifically in the evolution of the clinician's role in the <u>medical treatment system</u>. It's time for us to steer that change toward well-being for everyone.

Sincerely,
Anoop Kumar, MD, MM

CHAPTER 16
A Declaration of Well-Being

The word *radical* is derived from the word *root*. Radical action goes to the root of all action—you. It is action *you* take that changes *you*, and in so doing, it changes the situation around you. Radical action in health begins with contemplating the personal aspect of the big questions woven throughout this book.

What does well-being mean to me?
How can I be well?
How well do I know myself?

I invite you to consider these questions and use them as a launching pad to explore your own Three Bodies. The experience that awaits you is radically practical. It's practical because experiencing your Three Bodies marks the beginning of a profound level of self-care. It marks the beginning of unlocking the ability to begin healing chronic stress, chronic pain, and chronically suppressed and repressed emotions, which are among the root causes of many diseases. The possibilities for healing are endless.

Self-care will cause radical changes in the medical treatment system. The primary site of health care will shift from hospitals and clinics to wherever you happen to be—home, work, or at the ballgame. *The most powerful technology will be recognized as inner technology, free and always available*, to which the external technology currently being developed will be a perfect complement. This is the disruption that the old medical treatment system fears most, but its arrival is imminent. It starts with shifting your experience through action.

Throughout this book, I used personal stories and concepts to build a bridge between the medical treatment system and a true health care system. But stories and concepts are not effective if they remain just that. They are pointers to action, exploration, and experience. Below, I have summarized the key points in this book in A Declaration of Well-Being. I encourage you to visit anoopkumar.com to sign this declaration as an individual or organization as a first step to action.

A Declaration of Well-Being

- Our goal is well-being, not just better medical treatment. Well-being is the goal of a true health care system.
- Well-being connects individuals, families, communities, organizations, and our planet. Disease at any one of these levels affects the entire system.
- We have Three Bodies—Physical, Mental, and Energetic. Well-being is the state of balance among The Three Bodies, anchored in *being*.
- Principles of well-being and healing are universal. A complete Science of Well-Being reflects this understanding and codifies the principles that are common to every healing system.
- The most pervasive problem in the medical treatment system is the Informational Problem: medical science's understanding of the human being is remarkably incomplete.
- Developing a Science of Well-Being requires a more comprehensive understanding of energy, information, and consciousness. Such an understanding will provide a scientific framework within which to integrate medical science, all healing systems, and the digital revolution in medical care.
- Medical education and clinical care must become interprofessional. Tomorrow's health care leaders and clinicians must understand the strengths of each healing system and how to coordinate care among them. The integrative medicine movement is leading the way.
- Learning and working environments for clinical staff must be designed in accordance with the Blueprint for Well-Being. A

clinician experiencing well-being is ideally suited to help another heal and be well.
- An observer-based science is the next step in the evolution of science. Consciousness is at the core of an observer-based science. Today's objective science is a subset of observer-based science.

Visit anoopkumar.com to sign this declaration and find links to organizations that are already making this vision a reality. If you would like to recommend an organization to be added to the list, you may do so on the website.

Visit anoopkumar.com

CHAPTER 17
A Blueprint for Well-Being

When it comes to well-being, everything matters. Connection, nutrition, movement, and rest matter, as I addressed with The Four Pillars of well-being. The places we go matter, the thoughts we entertain matter, and our creative expression matters. In short, everything matters. That doesn't mean we should be paranoid about every action, mulling over whether what we are doing is right or wrong. Rather, it means that our ability to shape our lives is powerful, more powerful than it appears at first glance.

In the next few seconds, if you slow down your breathing and take deeper breaths, the state of your mind will change. Because the state of your mind changes, the way you experience and respond to the environment around you will also change. That's real power. If that much power can be summoned in a few seconds, imagine what can be accomplished with regular practice, when every action begins with greater awareness, understanding, and power.

We are inextricably connected with our surroundings. We are influencing them with every action, and they, in turn, influence us. This comprehensive vision is missing in the popular definition of well-being. In our society, transportation, housing, social connection, and so many other areas of life are generally not equated with well-being. Such connections are left to be developed by those in formal positions, such as public health officials, counselors, and social workers. But they can't do it by themselves. There's simply too much to integrate.

We are all invested in our well-being from the moment we wake up to the moment we sleep. It is important to bring all of these aspects of well-being together in one representation that will help us *design* well-being.

If Apple can design the revolutionary iPhone and Tesla can design the Model S, why can't we design well-being? We surely can.

This idea is the motivating factor behind the Blueprint for Well-Being, which applies The Four Pillars to each of The Three Bodies discussed in this book. This blueprint represents every aspect of well-being and can be used to design well-being at every level—individual, community, organization, society, and globe.

	CONNECTION	NUTRITION	MOVEMENT	REST
EXTENDED PHYSICAL BODY	Being in a setting you enjoy	Developing principles and practices of healthy community design, nurturing environments, ergonomic design, and sustainability.	Constructing and renovating spaces to reflect latest principles and practices (see Nutrition)	Maintaining environments appropriately; sustainable agriculture; restful spaces such as parks
PERSONAL PHYSICAL BODY	Recognizing biological cues and responding accordingly (i.e., hunger, need for a restroom, fatigue, pain)	More fresh, whole foods. Fewer processed foods. Less sugar and salt.	Breathing, stretching, yoga, walking jogging, sports, weight training	Sleep, massage, down time
MENTAL BODY	Meditation, conscious breathing	Reflection, contemplation, creative thinking, exposure to new ideas and experiences, engaging in dialogue	Creative expression of intuition, thoughts, and emotions to others; music and arts	Equanimity, meditation, sleep

ENERGETIC BODY	Recognizing the Energetic Body	Sustaining attention on the Energetic Body	Allowing the energy to flow unimpeded (couples with conscious breathing)	Remaining balanced in the Energetic Body

Across the top are The Four Pillars—connection, nutrition, movement, and rest. Each pillar is applied to a particular body—the extended Physical Body, the personal Physical Body, the Mental Body, and the Energetic Body—which are listed vertically along the left side. As an example, nutrition can apply to the Mental Body, in which case it applies to the kinds of thoughts that feed the mind.

This Blueprint for Well-Being can be used by individuals, communities, and organizations to answer a simple question: Are we doing our part to foster well-being for the people we care about? The medical treatment system in particular should implement the ideas in this blueprint to align medical training and treatment with well-being, rather than keeping them at odds. Each of us has a role to play in designing our Three Bodies in such a way that well-being flourishes on the personal, organizational, societal, and global scale. In doing so, we will co-design a masterpiece that even Michelangelo would envy.

Visit anoopkumar.com to see examples of how the Blueprint for Well-being can be applied.

GLOSSARY

<u>Allopathy</u>: A term coined by Samuel Hahnemann (the creator of homeopathy) to distinguish between two different approaches to medical treatment. The root *allo* means *other*. <u>Allopathy</u> therefore refers to a <u>healing system</u> in which the medicine given is generally *other than* or in opposition to the symptoms of illness, rather than primarily in support of the body's immune system.

<u>Anatomy</u>: A systematic way of drawing boundaries. The boundaries that are drawn depend on the vision and assumptions of the anatomist.

<u>Being</u>: The state prior to thinking, feeling, and doing. The state that is fundamental to experiences, including thinking, feeling, and doing. (See *Consciousness*.)

<u>Consciousness</u>: There are many subtypes of consciousness, such as waking, dreaming, human, animal, preconsciousness, and subconsciousness. Consciousness itself is more fundamental than all these subtypes. It is that which makes any and all experience possible, including the experiences of our lives, space, time, energy, and information. One description of consciousness is *limitless awareness*. Another word for consciousness is *being*. (See *Being*.)

<u>Energy</u>: The activity of consciousness. This activity can be experienced subjectively and partially measured objectively. Energy is always paired with information. Energy can be said to be the activity of information, or active information.

<u>Four Pillars, The</u>: Four areas of life that are central to cultivating well-being: connection, nutrition, movement, rest. The Four Pillars can be applied to each of <u>The Three Bodies.</u>

<u>Healing system</u>: A unique system of diagnosis and healing that understands and engages the many dimensions of a person's well-being. <u>Healing systems</u> are influenced by the culture in which they develop, and often

reflect different perspectives on human anatomy and physiology. The systematized form of allopathy we see today is more a medical treatment system than a healing system, but at times I refer to it as the allopathic healing system because of its inherent potential to become a complete system by further developing its science and aligning with other healing systems.

Health: Popularly defined as the state of balance and full functionality of the Physical Body. The World Health Organization defined health as more than a physical phenomenon, but in order to reflect how popular culture and medical science view health, as well as accommodate distinct concepts of wellness and well-being, I have defined it in terms of the Physical Body here. (See *Wellness* and *Well-being*.)

Health care system: The operationalized form of a healing system. Today's medical treatment system cannot be called a health care system because its science doesn't understand what health is or what care is, due to the limitations of objective science.

Information: A specific pattern of consciousness. Information is inseparable from energy. Energy is the active aspect of information.

Informational Problem: The current perspective in medical science that assumes the human being is primarily a Physical Body. This perspective has less appreciation of the Mental Body and little to no appreciation of the Energetic Body.

Integrative medicine: An interprofessional model of clinical practice in which every effective healing system has a place. Integrative medicine is the standard-bearer of a true health care system.

Introspective methods: Techniques for looking inward beyond the personal Physical Body to the Mental Body, Energetic Body, and *being*. Such methods include reflection, contemplation, and meditation.

Medical treatment system: A system that *treats* a person prior to understanding and engaging the many dimensions of that person's wellbeing.

The gap between *treatment* and *healing* is the gap between a medical treatment system and a healing system. When a medical treatment system realizes its full potential, it becomes a healing system. Thus, every medical treatment system is a healing system in the making.

Normal science: The activity of science that happens within an accepted and often unexamined paradigm. Science is interpreted through certain assumptions—for example, that the "external" world is independent of us, or that "solid" objects are fundamentally different than mental experiences. Such assumptions influence what we can understand from the data we collect, limiting understanding to what can be accepted as "normal."

Objective science: The type of science that studies an aspect of the universe as external and independent of the method of observation. It provides a useful, yet incomplete understanding of our reality. The word *objective* in this phrase is often misinterpreted to mean "free of bias," whereas it more precisely refers to the tendency to *objectify* what the scientist is studying as external and independent. In fact, objective science is always *subjectively interpreted* in the context of human thought and a human nervous system. Because of these inherent limitations, an objective-only science cannot fully comprehend or engage The Three Bodies, and therefore cannot be the sole foundation of a true health care system.

Observer-based science: A science that recognizes the universe is a subjective experience in consciousness, not an independent externality. Nothing can be studied independent of consciousness, because there would be no way to recognize or engage it. Observer-based science recognizes that the universe's appearance depends on the way we observe it. Such a science embraces the fact that subjectivity is inherent in apparent objectivity. Developing our understanding of this type of science is key to understanding The Three Bodies, engaging well-being, and developing a true health care system. Observer-based science may also be called subjective science or qualia science.

Science: A system of thought defined by observing, hypothesizing, and experimenting for the purpose of drawing conclusions about the universe and ourselves. (See *Normal science, Objective science, Observer-based science.*)

Science of Well-Being: A science that recognizes the full scope of the human being: all Three Bodies and consciousness. A Science of Well-Being will have a more complete understanding of energy, information, and consciousness.

Three Bodies, The: A representation of the human being as three distinct, experienceable bodies: Physical, Mental, and Energetic.

Well-being: The state of balance in the Physical, Mental, and Energetic Bodies, anchored in *being*. (See *Being*.)

Wellness: The state of balance in the Physical and Mental Bodies.